SOUTHERN GARDENER
AND RECEIPT BOOK

THE
SOUTHERN
GARDENER
AND RECEIPT BOOK

CONTAINING

DIRECTIONS FOR GARDENING;

A COLLECTION OF VALUABLE RECEIPTS FOR COOKERY, THE
PRESERVATION OF FRUITS AND OTHER ARTICLES OF
HOUSEHOLD CONSUMPTION, AND FOR THE
CURE OF DISEASES.

BY P. THORNTON,
OF CAMDEN, SOUTH CAROLINA.

Second Edition, Improved and Enlarged.

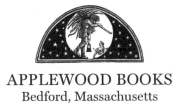

APPLEWOOD BOOKS
Bedford, Massachusetts

The second edition of *The Southern Gardener and Reciept Book* was originally printed in 1845.

Thank you for purchasing an Applewood book. Applewood reprints America's lively classics—books from the past that are still of interest to modern readers. For a free copy of our current catalog, write to:

Applewood Books
PO Box 365
Bedford, MA 01730

ISBN 1-55709-191-9

PREFACE.

Being the proprietor of a gardening establishment, I receive my seeds from persons who raise them, and others who may be confided in; therefore, I have no hesitation in saying they are always fresh and genuine. As there are sometimes complaints made that certain seeds will not vegetate, it may be well to give them a fair trial before they are condemned. Those that are good may sometimes fail of coming up, in various ways; some kinds may be sown too soon, and be chilled in the ground before they vegetate; at other times they may be scorched in the ground by the burning rays of the sun, are many times eaten up by insects, and very often are too deeply covered in the earth. All small seeds may be tried by putting them in water, and stirring them well. After standing a few minutes, those that are fresh and good will sink to the bottom. But the best way to prove them is by sowing a few in a small pot or box of light loose earth, and placing it in a warm room, exposed to the sun, and attending to keeping the earth moist. If the seed is good, it will vegetate in a reasonable time. Peas and beans may be tried by planting a few in the open ground before the time for planting a general crop. Although the proprietor is satisfied that his seeds are good before exposing them for sale, he would be glad that every person would try them as directed before they crop the ground. If the seeds do not grow, after being tried as above, they may be returned, and he will replace them with others or refund the money. The bug holes frequently seen in peas are not occasioned by age, but are the work of an insect which deposites its eggs in the flower, and matures with the pea, when it eats its way out at the side, leaving the eye of the pea uninjured—of course does not prevent its vegetation. Most of the complaints received of seeds not growing (particularly in the spring and summer months), are owing to their not being well rolled or pressed. Sowing on a large scale, rolling would be more expeditious; but for small sowings, the following may answer as a substitute :—

After the seed is sown, and the ground raked evenly, take a board, (of the whole length of the bed;) lay it flat on the ground, beginning at one end of the bed, walking the whole length of the board. This will press the soil on the seed. Then shift the board till you have thus gone over the whole bed. In dry, warm weather, cover your seed beds for two or three days with boards laid flat on the soil, or green pine boughs, taking care to remove them at night that they may have air and the night dew. By this method the seed will soon vegetate and grow. Late in the spring or summer months, seeds should not be sown or planted, unless there be a good season of rain, or that the ground be sufficiently moist. In a dry time the ground might be well watered over night, and sow or plant the following morning. In this case the seeds should be previously soaked in soft rain-water from thirty-six to forty-eight hours, particularly beets, as they are difficult to get up when sown late in the season, on account of the hard shell or covering. Therefore they should have forty-eight hours' soaking, letting them stand in the sun to keep the water warm. Parsnips or carrots might be soaked the same length of time.

VEGETATION OF GARDEN SEEDS.

The number of years different Garden Seeds will Vegetate.

	Years.		Years.
Artichoke	3	Horse Raddish	4
Asparagus	4	Hyssop	6
Balm	2	Jerusalem Artichoke	3
Basil	2	Lavender	2
Bean	1	Leek	2
Beet	10	Lettuce	3
Borage	4	Marigold	2
Broccoli	4	Melon	10
Burnet	6	Mint	4
Cabbage	4	Mustard	4
Calabash	7	Mangel wurzel	10
Camomile	2	Majoram	4
Caraway	4	Nasturtium	2
Carrot	1	Onion	2
Cauliflower	4	Parsley	6
Celery	10	Parsnip	1
Chervil	6	Pea	1
Cives	3	Pennyroyal	2
Corn	3	Potatoe	3
Corn Salad	2	Pumpkin	10
Coriander	3	Purslain	2
Cress	2	Radish	2
Cucumber	10	Rampion	2
Dandelion	10	Rape	4
Dock	1	Rhubarb	1
Endive	4	Rosemary	3
Fennel	5	Rue	3
Garlick	3	Ruta Baga	4
Gourd	10	Salsify	2
Hop	2	Samphire	3

	Years.		Years.
Summer Savory	2	Tansy	3
Scorzenera	2	Tarragon	4
Shalot	4	Thyme	2
Skirret	4	Tomato	2
Sorrel	7	Turnip	4
Spinach	4	Wormwood	2
Squash	10		

GERMINATION OF GARDEN SEED.

"M. Humboldt has made several experiments on the subject of the Germination of seeds in the oxymuriatic acid, or oxalic acid, diluted with water, and has found that this acid has a remarkable effect in accelerating the progress of vegetation. Cress seed, when thrown into the fluid at the temperature of 88° showed germs in three hours, while none were seen in water in twenty-six hours. Professor Pohl, at Dresden, produced in this manner, vegetation from dried seeds one hundred years' old; and Messrs. Jacquire and Vander Schott, at Vienna, have caused the growth of old seeds in the botanical garden, which have resisted every other method."

TO SAVE SEEDS.

From the Southern Agriculturist.

All seeds keep better in their seed vessels, but this can rarely be done, on account of the great space occupied. As soon, therefore, as the pods of cabbages, turnips, radishes, &c., turn brown and a part become dry, the stems should be cut and laid on a cloth or floor to dry, afterwards thrashed out, and hung up in bags in some open airy place. Lettuces should be pulled up by the roots, as soon as there is the least appearance of maturity, and hung up, and the plants will ripen all their seeds, nearly at the same time. If left in the garden to ripen, the earliest and best will be lost; in fact, except under very favorable circumstances, very few will be obtained, as every shower and every strong breeze will lessen the quantity, and scatter those which are mature over the whole garden. The same course should be pursued with leeks and onions.—It is a prevalent opinion that the bush squash cannot be perpetuated among us, as such have a strong tendency to run, and will in one or two seasons become a vine. This is a mistake, and originated, no doubt, in the manner of saving the seed. If the first squashes which appear be retained for seed, there is no danger of the plant running the next season; but if these be used, and those which are borne at the extremes are preserved for this purpose, they will run, and moreover be later in bearing. To have early fruit of either squashes, cucumbers or mellons, the very first should be reserved.

INSTRUCTIONS

FOR

WORKING A KITCHEN GARDEN.

ALPHABETICALLY ARRANGED.

THE TIME FOR SOWING AND PLANTING IS CALCTLATED TO ANSWER FOR CAMDEN AND THE ADJACENT COUNTRY FOR FORTY OR FIFTY MILES, BUT IN A SOUTH-WEST DIRECTION, IT MAY ANSWER THROUH THE WHOLE STATE OF GEORGIA AND ALABAMA.

DIRECTIONS FOR GARDENING.

ASPARAGUS

May be sown any time during the month of March, in a small bed of light, rich soil, drilled in rows nine inches apart, which would be preferable to broad cast, on account of hoeing and keeping them clear of weeds, covering them one inch deep; should the weather prove dry, water them occasionally. In twelve months (or say in the month of February, after the plants are up), they may be set out in beds six feet wide, by twenty-five or thirty feet in length, with walks or alleys two-and-a-half feet wide between each bed, sufficient to admit a wheelbarrow. The beds are previously prepared by spading to the depth of twelve or fifteen inches. After the bed is levelled and raked fine, proceed to lay it off in trenches, across the bed, two feet apart from each other, each trench to be dug fifteen inches wide and two-and-a-half feet deep, laying up the soil in ridges between each trench. Should the natural soil not be good to that depth, the inferior at the bottom may be removed and carried off. after this is done, throw in eighteen inches of well rotted stable manure; after levelling the same, add two inches of soil on the manure, taken from the sides which were thrown out of the ridges; level this also and rake it finely, and all is ready for planting.

Then be careful in selecting such plants only as have good fibres, and a fine bold crown; in setting out, place them eighteen inches apart, and lay out the fibres in regular order, and not tumble them together, as is too often done, to the great injury of the plants. When this is done, cover them with two inches more of the soil from the sides of the ridges as before, and the work is done. Plants eighteen months or two years' old would be preferable, as they would be more vigorous. The plants throughout the summer must be kept clear of weeds, and occasionally hoed, and the loose dirt gradually thrown in from the sides of the ridges. By these operations, and the summer rains, the trenches will by October be filled up as level as the bed was before setting out the roots. Upon the approach of cold weather, and after the tops have been killed by frost, they should be cut down even with the ground and carried off; the bed should then be covered with two or three inches of coarse stable manure, partly rotten, which should remain on the bed until spring, when it must be forked, or hoed carefully into the surface of the bed so as not to injure the crowns of the roots. Just before the shoots make their appearance in the spring, the beds should be carefully raked free from weeds.

Vegetable seed of any description should not be sown in the beds between the plants, as it exhausts the goodness of the soil. The first year after planting the bed, a few of the strongest shoots may be cut, but it should be sparingly, as the roots will be all the better afterward. Continue to pursue the same system of culture every year, and the roots will rapidly increase in vigor. Beds prepared in this manner, and yearly attended to, will last many years, and the produce will be of a superior quality. Asparagus thrives in a light, rich soil, neither too wet nor too dry. There are two or three varieties of this plant, but the giant asparagus is the largest and most productive.

ARTICHOKE.

This is a perennial plant, a fine vegetable for table use, and highly esteemed by many. There are two or three varieties. The largest globe has a dusky, purplish head; the dwarfish globe is a prolific variety, and valuable as occupying less room with its head. They are propagated by suckers, or by seed. The seed may be sown any time during the month of March, in small beds of tolerably light, good soil, drilled in rows twelve inches apart. In order to procure good thrifty plants, the seeds should be dropped singly nine or ten inches apart, and covered two inches deep; work them occasionally, keeping the ground loose and light, and free from weeds. About the last of August, or early in September, the plants may be set out in large beds of a deep rich light soil, moist but not wet, giving the plants three feet space each way, being careful that the hearts do not get covered with the earth. It would be well to have the beds situated so as to have a gentle slope, sufficient to carry off any superfluous moisture or water that might accumulate during the winter or spring. If the slope of the beds were to face the south, it might hasten the vegetation of the plants so as to produce heads for use the following summer. Late in the fall, or about the last of November, when vegetation has ceased, the dead leaves may be removed from the plants, and the beds covered with a good coat of manure from the stable, partly rotten, with fine straw, or other coarse litter, to the depth of two or three inches, observing that the plants be lightly covered. In the spring, before the plants begin to vegetate, the beds may be lightly spaded, or hoed, so as not to injure the plants, and raked finely afterward, in order to destroy all superfluous weeds. The ground should be worked occasionally during the spring and summer, so as to be kept light and loose, and free from weeds. By the above mode and treatment, the plants will bear and do well for six or seven years. After the plants have been bearing two years, the stocks may be examined in the spring (say the last of February), and two or three of the strongest or best shoots being selected for growing, the rest are removed with a knife or chisel. These shoots or suckers may be transplanted into new beds, as before described. When all the heads from a stem are taken, cut off the stem close to the ground, to give the plant more strength for new shoots.

The plant called Jerusalem artichoke is not properly an artichoke, and would not be ranked as a vegetable for the table. Its root, which is similar to a potatoe, contains but very little nutriment, therefore is but of little value. The growth of the plant or stalk resembles the sunflower, and is of the easiest possible cultivation; will grow in almost any soil, and when it has once got possession of the ground it is very difficult to eradicate: as hogs will eat them, they are sometimes cultivated for that purpose. For a crop, they may be planted after the ground is well ploughed, any time in March, in drills two and a half or three feet apart, and may be planted and worked as corn crops, hilling them a little when worked with a hoe. They may be cut in two or three pieces like potatoes, and dropped in the drills twelve inches apart, and covered two or three inches deep. They will produce more abundantly in a strong light clay soil. As the root is firm and hard, they are sometimes made use of for pickles.

BEETS

May be sown the last of February, or early in March, and in order for a succession of crops, they may be sown till the last of April, in beds prepared of a light, strong, rich soil, and spaded to the depth of twelve or fifteen inches, and made four or five feet wide. After the beds are levelled and raked finely, they may be drilled in rows, twenty inches apart. The seeds may be dropped singly five or six inches apart, and covered two inches deep. As the plants will admit, thin out to stand singly twelve or fifteen inches apart. In order to have large thrifty plants, the ground should be frequently worked, and made very light and loose, and kept free from weeds. Should the fall season prove favorable by not being dry, they might be sown from the first to the tenth of August, and come to perfection before the winter sets in; but the early sowing is most favorable to this climate. Beets sown in a light dry soil, after the month of March, should be soaked thirty-six hours, and kept in the sun in the course of the day, to keep the water warm; after the seeds are sown and raked in, the ground should be well pressed. When the beets have got their growth, which may be noted by the top being decayed or become dead, they may be dug up, and preserved by packing them away in light dry sand, either in boxes or barrels. It would be well to spread them on the ground for a day or two, in the shade, to give them air to evaporate the surplus moisture.

BEANS.

Bush beans of all descriptions, if the spring be favorable, may be planted the first of April, and in order for a succession of crops, they should be planted once in two or three weeks till the last of May, in a light rich soil, in trenches from two to two-and-a-half feet apart, covered two inches; and when the plants will admit, hoe and thin them out to stand four or five inches apart. Bush beans, for a full crop, may be planted from the fifteenth of July to the twentieth of August. Pole beans, of all descriptions, may be planted from the fifth of April to the last of May, in drills from three to five feet apart, according to the height they run; and as the plants will admit, thin them out to stand from nine to twelve inches apart. Two beans or vines may be admitted to run to one pole. Sometimes they are planted in hills from three to four feet apart each way, and three or four beans may be planted in a hill, but only two thrifty vines left to run to one pole. Those kinds which do not run so much, may be planted with corn when about six inches in height, and if the soil be light and strong, will do well; but when this method is adopted, the corn should be planted in drills or trenches from four to five feet apart, and the corn thinned out to stand two feet apart between each stalk. Then plant two or three to each stalk, leaving only two or three thrifty plants to run. Lima beans might be planted with advantage in a single row, along a border on each side of a walk, and poles might be bent over in the form of an arch for them to run on. By this means they might be easily gathered when grown. They are one of the best kind of shell beans for table use, and require a good strong light soil. They will bear till frost, and will stand the dry weather much better than any other kind. They are, therefore, the most profitable crop. They may be gathered in the fall, after they become dry, and laid away for winter use. By soaking them in soft water over night, previous to cooking them, they will boil very sweet and tender, and they are fine for soup. As they are more tender than other varieties, they should not be planted sooner than the tenth or fifteenth of April. Windsor beans are one of those varieties that are very hardy, and will stand the winter frost. For early spring use, they may be planted from the first to the middle of October, in a strong rich soil, in trenches from two and a half to three feet apart, and covered three inches deep; and when the plants will admit, they may be thinned out so as to stand from six to eight inches apart, and for a succession of crops they might be planted again the last of February and early in March.

BORECOLE.

Is a species of cabbage, and one of those hardy plants, the leaves of which may be cut without injury to its growth, and will produce a new crop in the course of a month or six weeks. They may be sown in small beds, made light and loose, about the last of February, or any time during the month of March, in drills nine inches apart, and covered one inch deep. In order to have good thrifty plants, and of a regular size, thin them out a little soon after they are up, and in a few days more thin them out again, so as to give the plants three or four inches' space; and when the plants will admit, they may be set out in beds or squares previously dug, and made light and loose, at the distance of two-and-a-half feet apart each way. It should be observed that the land must be well manured, and in a high state of tillage, for the cultivation of this plant, which, if kept constantly hoed, will grow very luxuriantly, and in the hottest weather be infinitely more brittle in the leaves than any other kind cultivated in gardens, which is a certain indication of its being a healthy plant. It is worthy of the attention of the farmer or grazier on account of the rapidity of its growth and the property of withstanding the effect of severe frost, while it affords an excellent vegetable for the table, and may be used with advantage for feeding cows and sheep. There are several species of this plant, but the green curled borecole is the hardest and best.

BROCCOLI,

A species of cabbage cultivated for the use of the table. There are several kinds of this plant, but the purple Cape Broccoli is said to be the best. It may be sown about the latter end of February or early in March, in any tolerable soil, in drills eight or nine inches apart, and covered one inch deep; and when plants have germinated eight leaves, they should be transplanted into nursery beds, in rows twelve inches apart, and the plants five or six inches from each other. By this means the plants would have a more regular stout growth. Should the weather prove dry, they might be frequently watered, which should be done at night, observing to stir the ground loose around the plants the following morning; and in order to make them flourish and grow, they should be kept in a good state of tillage, and free from weeds during the whole growth. About the first of May they may be set out in large beds of a light strong soil, and well sheltered, or where the shade would strike them early in the day, giving them a few hours of the early morning sun: give the plants two feet space from each other. As our summers frequently prove too hot and dry for the early sowing and planting of this vegetable to mature and come to perfection, they might be sown about the middle of July, on shady beds or borders, and watered occasionally should the weather prove dry, observing when the plants are well up to thin them out six or eight inches apart, to give them a good regular growth; and about the middle of August they might be set out in beds, as above described. They would then be apt to flower and head well before the hard weather set in. Should the winter prove mild, they would continue to head and put out during the winter season.

CAULIFLOWER.

The early cauliflower may be sown from the tenth to the last of February, in any tolerable soil, in drills six inches apart, and covered one inch deep: and when they produce three leaves they may be put into nursery beds, as the broccoli, and about the last of April set out or transplanted, where they may remain, giving them a good light soil. The late cauliflower may be sown about the last of April, and set out in nursery beds as above; and about the last of June, they may be set out where they are to remain, giving them a space of two feet each way. Those that are headed must have the heads shaded by breaking the large leaves over them.

CARROTS,

For summer use, may be sown from the middle of February to the last of March, in beds prepared four feet wide, of a light rich soil, drilled in rows twelve inches apart, and covered one inch deep. As soon as the plants are well up, they may be thinned out, to stand one or two inches apart, and as they advance a little in size, thin them out to stand three or four inches from each other. By this mode, and frequently stirring the ground finely, the roots will be of a regular and good size. For winter and spring use, carrots may be sown from the first to the last of August, and treated as above.

NOTE. Carrots should not be sown late in the

spring, and early in the fall, unless there be a good season of rain, observing to roll or press the ground after the seeds are raked in.

EARLY CABBAGE

May be sown the last of January, or early in February, in warm beds of any tolerably light soil, either in broad cast, or in drills nine inches apart, which would be preferable, on account of hoeing and keeping them free from weeds: cover them one inch deep, and when the plants are well up, they may be thinned out to stand two or three inches apart. By this means they will be more thrifty, and regular in size. When the plants will admit, they may be set out in beds of rich mould, previously made loose and light, each plant two feet apart.

Late cabbage may be sown the last of May, or any time in June, and remain in the beds till August before transplanting, and may be set out in the same manner as the early ones.

Green glazed cabbage may be sown any time in February or March, and treated as the others, only giving them a little more space when transplanted. Early cabbage, sown from the twentieth of September, to the first of October, on a warm border, would produce heads two or three weeks earlier, should the winter prove favorable, and not too severe.

RAISING CABBAGES FROM CUTTINGS.
From the Vermont Chronicle.

A neighbor of ours tells us, that he, accidentally, raised some fine cabbages from cuttings last year. Some pieces of old stumps happened to be buried in the spring, at the proper depth. They soon sent up shoots (one each) at an early day, and formed excellent heads. There was no tendency to seed, any more than from plants obtained in the usual way.

To try the experiment of getting early cabbages in this way, cut the stump into small pieces, with one bud on each; plant and cultivate them as you would plants from the seed.

TO KILL LICE ON CABBAGE.

Last year I had one quarter of an acre of cabbages that were nearly covered with the cabbage louse. I took off the outside leaves, and burned them. Having a few gallons of very strong tobacco liquor (left after sheep-shearing,) which I diluted by adding soap-suds from the wash, I sprinkled the plants very thoroughly from a watering pot. I believe it killed every louse, for I did not discover one afterwards.

New England Farmer.

TO DESTROY WORMS ON CABBAGE.

Tobacco leaves strewn upon and among cabbages are said to be effectual in preventing the ravages of cabbage worms.

SOLID CELERY

May be sown in March, on a small bed of light rich soil, in drills six or nine inches apart, and covered lightly. When the plants are up to the height of an inch or two, they may be thinned out to stand three or four inches apart, so as to give them a regular, good growth. Should the weather prove dry, the plants may be occasionally watered at night, observing to stir the ground between the plants the following morning. When the plants are from six to nine inches in height, and have acquired a stocky growth, they may be set out in a very rich moist soil, previously prepared, in trenches three feet apart and a spade deep : lay the earth on each side of the trenches, and dig the bottom, leaving them level: place the plants along the trenches upright six inches apart, and water them, should the weather prove dry afterwards ; they might be shaded in the day for two or three days till they have taken root. In three or four weeks draw the earth to each side of the plants, breaking it fine : do this in dry weather, and be careful not to bury the hearts: repeat the earthing once in ten or twelve days till the plants are fit for use. In order for a succession of crops they may be sown in April and May, and treated as above. Seeds sown later than April should be sown in a moist shady situation, and the ground well pressed : as they are sometimes difficult to get up when sown late, it might be well to water the beds for three or four evenings, should the weather prove dry, and cover them in the day with green pine boughs.

CURLED CRESS OR PEPPERGRASS

May be sown the last of March, or early in April, in beds of a tolerably good soil, in drills six inches apart, and covered lightly; and in order for a succession of crops it may be sown once in two or three weeks till the last of May.

Garden cress may be sown as above, only give it nine inches space between the drills, and as soon as well up thin them out so that the plants may stand single two or three inches apart.

CUCUMBERS

For early use, may be planted about the first of April, in a good, warm, light soil: should the nights prove cool about the time they should come up, or after, the hills may be covered with straw at night, and removed in the day when the sun is up so as to warm the hills. For a succession of crops, the long green may be planted for pickling the last of May, and early in June, in a moist soil, so it be light and good; the early sort in hills four feet apart each way; and the long green, or late sort, in hills six feet apart each way, leaving only one thrifty plant in a hill to grow. Put no fresh manure in the hills, as it is too powerful, and will cause them to wilt and die. If the soil be light and poor, make up hills about two feet square, by throwing out the soil to the depth of fifteen or eighteen inches; then fill up the hole with good rich mould, well pulverized; a little of the top soil first taken off might be mixed with the mould near the top, observing to leave the hill only a little above the level of the ground. In order that they may be kept in a flourishing state, and bear till late, the ground must be kept loose and free from weeds, and no cucumber suffered to remain on the vine till full grown, unless they be such as are wanting for seed. Should the weather prove very dry, they might be occasionally watered at night, by digging a small trench round near the hills before the vines commence running; fill it up with water that it may evaporate to the roots, which is a preferable mode to sprinkling the water on the tops of the hills, or plants, as vines are very tender. The seeds should not be planted till the ground is warm; they will then come up quick, and grow without any obstruction; otherwise, if they come up, and get stunted by the cold, they do not flourish well afterwards. For a fall crop for pickling, they might be planted the last of July, and early in August. To save cucumbers from the streaked bug, plant an onion in each hill.

NOTE. When cucumbers are planted later than the month of April, it would be well to spread a coat of fine straw on the ground between the hills to the depth of three or four inches, put on after a rain while it is wet. By this method they would not suffer by the drought; and if the season prove wet, the vines will not be so liable to rot.

NOVEL METHOD OF RAISING CUCUMBERS.

After all that Gulliver and the doctors have said against cucumbers, they are still a welcome dish upon most tables, and when eaten in moderation are probably healthful. That they are not so when eaten immoderately is, we have no doubt, also true. Cucumbers are most sought after early in the season, and we have picked up our pen to tell how we managed last year to have them in perfection long before they were plentiful in market.

Having cleared the soil to the depth of twelve or fifteen inches from a space four feet in diameter, we placed an old nail-keg in the centre, and filled up around with fresh manure, and covered it over with six or eight inches of earth, forming a mound of a foot or more in height, and six feet in diameter, with the open-ended keg in the centre, into which in very dry weather we could pour water, which would escape into the manure through the openings, and prevent the perishing of the vines. The seeds were planted in the mound (not in the keg, for that was empty) in March or in April, and the heat of the fermenting manure forced them vigorously. We had heavy frost afterward, and the surface of the earth was completely frozen; but it was only necessary to lay a board over the plants, and the warmth below was amply sufficient to protect them. The only object in using the keg was to prevent the water from running off and forming gutters down the sides of the mound. The plan worked well, and as it is now about time to renew the experiment, we publish it that others also may enjoy the advantages. A frame for the vines to run upon is advantageous.—*Germantown Telegraph.*

EGG PLANT

May be sown on a warm border about the first of April, in drills nine inches apart, and covered one inch deep; and where the plants will admit, they may be set out in beds of a light rich soil, giving them two feet space each way between the plants; hoe, and keep them free from weeds, and as they advance in size draw a little earth round the stems. There are two varieties of this plant, the white and the purple: the latter is preferable for table use; the white is more for ornament, as the growth is not so large. The plants may be set out eighteen inches apart. They make a handsome ornament for the flower pot.

GHERKINS

May be planted from the middle of April to the last of May, in any tolerable soil, so that it is light and warm, in hills six or eight feet apart, leaving but one thrifty plant in a hill to grow. If they be kept free from weeds, and the summer is moderately dry, they will bear abundantly till frost. They are very fine for pickles.

GOURDS

May be planted from the first to the last of April, in a good, light, rich soil, in hills six or eight feet apart. And the mammoth gourd may be planted from the middle of March to the last of April, in hills from eight to ten feet apart.

KAIL,

For early spring greens, may be sown about the last of January, in small beds of a light rich soil, in drills twelve inches apart, and covered one inch deep. As soon as the plants are well up, thin them out to stand two or three inches apart: afterward they may be thinned out for use as they advance in size: those that remain for seed should have fifteen or eighteen inches space.

LETTUCE,

For early use, may be sown the last of January on warm borders of a light rich soil, prepared well and raked fine, in drills nine inches apart, and covered lightly; and in order that the plants may be fine, and of a regular size, thin them out as soon as they are well up, to stand three or four inches apart; stir the ground frequently, and keep them free from weeds. As soon as the plants will admit set them out in beds, or round the borders, fifteen inches apart; if the ground be very rich and light they will head well. In order for a succession they may be sown once in three or four weeks till the last of April.

LAVENDER, SAGE, BALM, TANSY, THYME, RUE, ROSEMARY, OR OTHER HERBS,

May be sown by the last of March, or early in April, in small beds made light and fine, and drilled in rows nine inches apart, and covered one inch deep. When the plants will admit they may be thinned out, to stand four or five inches apart: in the following winter, say January or February, they may be set out in small beds, each plant from eighteen inches to two feet apart, according to the size they grow.

MUSTARD,

For winter use, may be sown from the middle of September to the middle of October, on warm borders of a tolerably rich light soil, and covered lightly in drills fifteen inches apart; for spring use, it may be sown again from the middle to the last of February, in beds spaded and well prepared, in drills eighteen inches apart. In order that the plants may flourish and grow quick, thin them out as soon as they are well up, to stand two or three inches apart. Afterwards they may be thinned out as wanted for use. Those that are to remain for seed should be thinned out to stand twelve or fifteen inches apart.

NASTURTIUMS

May be sown the last of March, or early in April, in a very light rich soil, in drills four feet apart; drop the seeds three or four inches apart, and cover them two inches deep: when the plants will admit, thin them out, to stand nine inches apart. The plants should be supported from the ground by bushy sticks.

Should the spring be dry, they should be occasionally watered in the evening, observing to stir the ground around the roots loosely the following morning. In a warm climate they would flourish best planted on a shady border, where the shade would strike them early in the day. The leaves, as well as the fruit, are sometimes used for pickles. As it is very ornamental, they might be planted in boxes, with a light rich soil, one seed in a box, and watered every evening till they come up, and placed on a shelf on the shady side of the house. They should be watered every evening, if the weather be dry, and the ground loosened around the plant the following morning. By this method the plants will grow very luxuriantly.

OKRA

May be planted any time in the month of April, in a large bed of light rich soil, drilled in rows four feet apart, and covered one inch deep. When the plants will admit, thin them out, to stand one-and-a-half or two feet distant, according to the strength of the ground. If the okra be planted in drills, six feet apart, cucumbers might be planted in hills between the rows, and do very well.

ONIONS

May be sown by the middle, or the last of February, but, in this climate, the month of September would be best: and prepared in beds four feet wide, of old rotten dung, or any strong rich soil: the soil should not be too wet or stubborn. When the ground will rake easily they may be sown thinly in drills fifteen inches apart, and covered one inch deep. If the soil is light, roll or press the ground after the seed is covered, and then rake the beds. The after culture is very simple: it consists merely in keeping them free from weeds, and the soil kept light and loose, observing not to draw any earth up to the roots while growing. As soon as the plants are well up they should be thinned out, to stand two or three inches apart, and when the plants are large enough, they may afterward be thinned out for daily use till they have four or five inches space. Should any of those sown in the fall be inclined to go to seed, the buds should be nipped out. When the leaves wither and die, the onions should be gathered, which should be done in dry weather. Spread them on clear dry ground for a few days to harden, frequently turning them about; and after carefully cleaning them from the earth they may be spread on a floor, giving them air when the weather is dry. For a few weeks after that, they may be kept from the air, frequently turning them, and picking out any that may be injured, or they might be tied up in bunches, and hung up in some cool place.

Plant the best and largest onions for seeds the following spring, in drills or rows twelve inches apart, and six inches from each other in the drill; and let them be set so deep as to be covered over with earth about one inch. When their heads come out, support the stalks with a stake to each, and when the seed is ripe gather and dry it.

MODE OF RAISING ONIONS IN THE TOWN OF WETHERSFIELD, CONNECTICUT.

The town of Wethersfield has long been famous

for the large quantities of onions which are annually raised, and exported to the West Indies and the southern States. It has been superstitiously supposed that there is something in the soil of Wethersfield peculiarly adapted to the culture of onions; and this whim has, no doubt, discouraged many from attempting the cultivation of this valable root in other sections of the country equally favourable to its growth. It is true the soil of Wethersfield is a rich sandy loam, well adapted to horticultural purposes; but the success of its inhabitants in the cultivation of onions, is attributable in a much greater degree to a particular virtue in the fingers of its females, than any peculiar properties of its soil.

The business of raising onions in Wethersfield is reduced to a perfect system. The following is the method of cultivation. Early in the spring, the land is manured by ploughing in fine manure from the stable or barn-yard, in the proportion of about ten loads to the acre. That of neat cattle is preferred, as that of horses is considered of too heating a nature. After the manure is ploughed in, the land is well harrowed and laid out in beds five feet wide.

The beds are laid out by turning a furrow toward them each way. This raises the bed above the aisles, and gives an opportunity for the water to run off should there be occasion for it. They are then raked with an iron tooth or common hay rake, and the aisles suffered to remain as left by the plough. Thus prepared, the beds are ready to receive the seed.

As early as the season will admit the seed is sown in the following manner. A rake with teeth a foot apart is drawn crosswise to the beds, for the purpose of making drills for the reception of the seeds. The seed is then sown in the drills with the thumb and fingers, and covered with the hand. From ten to twelve pounds of seed is put upon an acre. After the plants come up they are kept free from weeds, which generally requires four weedings; a hoe of suitable width to pass between the rows is used in weeding, which saves much labor. When ripe, they are pulled, and the tops cut off with a knife. A sufficient length of top is left to tie them to the straw in roping, or in bunches of three and a half pounds, as required by a law of the State. An ordinary crop is from six thousand to eight thousand ropes to the acre. The quantity annually raised in the town is estimated from one million to two millions and a half of ropes, which are sold at an average price of two dollars a hundred, amounting to from twenty to thirty thousand dollars.

Most of the labor of raising onions in Wethersfield is performed by females. The cultivation of an acre requires from fifty to sixty days' labor of a female, whose wages, including board, is about forty-two cents a day. Though many of the young ladies of Wethersfield spend a portion of their time in their onion gardens, yet in personal beauty, education, and politeness, they are not excelled by females of far less industrious habits.

LEEKS

May be sown early in September on a warm border open to the south, in drills nine inches apart, and covered lightly. About the middle of February following, the plants may be drawn up and set out in beds of four or five feet wide, previously prepared by spading in rich manure well rotted and pulverized, and the beds may be laid off in trenches of four or five inches deep and fifteen inches apart. Make holes with a dibble three inches deep at the bottom of the rench, and six inches apart, to receive the roots. A portion of the straggling roots and tops may be cropped or cut off; and when the plants are set, close the dirt lightly around the roots, and leave the trench open, and draw up the earth to the plants as they grow till the trenches are made level. By this method the roots will be fine and well blanched.

PARSNIPS

May be sown about the last of February, or any time during the month of March, in beds prepared four feet wide, of a very rich light earth, dug at least a full spade deep, and drilled in rows eighteen inches apart, and covered one inch deep. When the plants will admit, they may be thinned out to stand twelve or fifteen inches apart. Cabbage seed may be drilled between each row, and do well, as they would be removed before they would prove an injury to the parsnips. Peppergrass might also be sown in drills between the parsnips, and would prove no injury, as it is made use off as salads, or rather used with lettuce, and would be removed before the parsnips got to be of any size.

NOTE.—As parsnips, carrots and beets, are difficult seed to get up when sown late, they should not be sown after the month of March, without a good season of rain, soaking the parsnips and carrots from twenty-four to thirty-six hours, and the beets forty-eight hours before planting, either in warm water or letting it stand in the sun, which will answer the purpose, observing to press the ground well after the seeds are sown and raked in; and if the soil is light and dry, it would be well, after the seed is raked in, to cover the bed a few days with plank or green pine bushes, observing to remove them at night to give the beds air, and to have the advantage of the night dews. By this method they will not fail to come up, if the seed is good.

PARSLEY

May be sown early in February, but would do best sown in September, in small beds of a good light soil, in drills six inches apart, and covered one inch deep. As soon as the plants will admit, thin them out to stand three or four inches apart. As parsley seed seldom vegetates under five or six weeks, it would be best to give it rather a shady border; and if sown after February, it would be advisable to soak the seed twelve hours in water, mixed with sulphur, observing to press the ground well after the seed is raked in; and should the weather prove dry afterwards, occasionally water the bed. By this method it would soon vegetate and come up.

PEPPERS

May be sown from the tenth to the last of April, in small beds of a light rich soil, thinly, in drills fifteen to eighteen inches apart, and covered one inch deep. As soon as the plants will admit, thin them out to stand twelve inches apart. Those plants that are drawn out may be transplanted into large beds, of a strong rich soil, giving them eighteen inches space each way.

ENGLISH PEAS,

For an early spring crop, may be planted any time in December in a light rich soil, drilled in rows four feet apart, and those that grow very tall require five feet space, covering them two inches deep. As the winter often proves too severe, they might do full as well, or better, planted the last of January, or early in February; and in order for a succession of crops, they may be planted once in three or four weeks after, till the middle of April. They have been proved to do full as well, or better, planted in ridges around the edges or borders of beds, which makes a great saving of ground, and are much easier gathered. It is a good plan to plant two rows together, about nine inches apart, so that by setting bushes between them they may hold up both rows. The ground should be frequently stirred and made fine around the roots, and kept free from weeds; and, as they advance in height, draw a little earth to the stems. Peas that do not require sticks may be planted in drills two and a half feet apart, or on the edges or borders of beds, as the other kind.

POTATOES

Planted from the middle of February to the middle of April, are raised with the greatest success in this climate: a later planting seldom turns out well, owing generally to the heat and dryness of summer. A light soil, which is neither too dry nor too wet, suits them best. The ground should be well ploughed once or twice previous to planting, and if the ground was ploughed late in the fall, to have the winter exposure, so much the better, in order that the ground might be made mellow and fine. After preparing the ground for planting, lay off the trenches three feet apart, seven or eight inches deep, and throw in the bottom coarse straw or litter from the stable, one or two inches thick, pressing it down evenly; and on this put a compost of stable and cow-pen manure, tolerably well rotted, to about the same thickness; then cut your potatoes, so that there may be one or two good eyes in each piece, from the middle of the potatoe, rejecting both ends, or what is called the eye or top of the potatoe, and the bottom or root end; then drop them in the trench nine inches apart, and cover them with the earth taken from the drill, three or four inches deep, taking care to have the ridge covered very little above the level of the ground. One good moulding will be sufficient, after the potatoes get about six or eight inches in height.

ANOTHER METHOD OF RAISING POTATOES.

From the Farmer's Gazette.

DATED AT CEDAR HILL, ANSON CO., N. C., AUG. 3, 1840.
DR. MCLEAN:

Dear Sir :—Some few weeks since I saw in the columns of your paper an account of some fine Irish potatoes presented to you by Mr. A. P. Lacoste, weighing from fourteen to sixteen ounces, and measuring from ten to eleven inches in circumference. My mode of raising them is as follows: The latter part of February, I make trenches about ten or twelve inches deep by running a plough two or three times in a place, and scraping them out with a hoe. In these trenches I put a small quantity of stable or other strong manure, drop the potatoe and fill the trenches with half rotted straw or trash from the woods or barnyard. I then level the ground, and scatter leaves or other trash, about four or five inches deep all over the surface, which keeps the ground moist, and prevents the weeds and grass from growing. I have no trouble in working them afterwards. I have tried different modes of raising potatoes, but this is much the best. If you think the above worthy of a place in the columns of the Farmer's Gazette, it is at your disposal.   D. C. LILLY.

RADISHES.

This root being liable to be eaten by worms, the following method is recommended for raising them. Take equal quantities of buckwheat-bran and fresh horse manure, and mix them well and plentifully, and spread a thick coat on the bed intended for sowing, and spade it in, so that it may get thoroughly mixed. Suddenly after this a great fermentation will be produced, and a number of toadstools (a kind of mushroom) will start up in forty-eight hours. Dig the ground over again, and sow the seeds in drills early in February, and when well up, they may be thinned out, regularly, to stand three or four inches apart, and keep the ground loose and free from weeds. By this method they will grow with great rapidity, and be free from insects. Buckwheat-bran is an excellent manure itself. A second crop of radishes might be raised on the same bed after the first is done, by spading up the ground, and sowing and managing as at first.—*Farmer's Assistant.*

RHUBARB, OR PIE PLANT,

May be propagated either by seed or cuttings: the

seeds may be sown on a warm bed early in March, in drills eighteen inches apart, and dropped thinly; and when well up and in a growing state, they may be thinned out, in order to give the plants a good regular growth, to stand six inches apart. The soil should be kept light and loose around the plants, and free from weeds during the summer: and in the month of September following, the plants may be removed to a stationary bed, previously prepared, of a deep rich mould, well spaded in, the ground inclined to be moist, but not wet. The plants may be set out two-and-a-half feet each way; and, before the cold weather sets in, there may be a coat of half rotted manure spread over the beds, which will benefit and strengthen the roots. The after management of rhubarb requires good culture, and keeping them clean; and every fall the beds should have a good coat of well rotted manure spread over. As young plants produce the most tender stalks or canes, new beds should be made once in three years, which might be done by dividing the old roots and crowns in such a manner that each set has one or more eyes, and planting in September, as above stated.

SALSIFY, OR VEGETABLE OYSTER,

Is a white root, resembling a parsnip, and may be sown in small beds, and cultivated in the same manner.

SHALLOTS

May be planted by the middle or the last of February, in drills about fifteen inches apart, laid open three or four inches deep, and in each drill put a sprinkling of salt evenly, and upon that a layer of dry soot, about half an inch thick; then plant the roots upon it, about six inches apart, and cover up the drill evenly, with the earth firmly round the roots; keep them free from weeds during their growth, and work the ground evenly, without drawing up the earth round the roots. By this method they will produce fine large bulbs.

SPINACH, OR SPINAGE,

For winter use, may be sown the last of September, and again in October; and in order to have a succession of crops for spring use, it may be sown again in February and early in March, in a light strong soil, drilled in rows fifteen inches apart, and covered one inch deep. As soon as the plants are well up, thin them out to stand three or four inches apart; afterward they may be thinned out for use as they advance in size. If any are left to remain for seed, they should have about fifteen inches space.

NEW-ZEALAND SPINAGE,

A new valuable sort, which may be planted from the twentieth of February to the last of March, in beds prepared, four feet wide, of a good, light, rich mould, in drills twenty inches apart, the seeds dropped singly six inches apart in the drill, and covered nearly two inches deep; and if they should all come up, the plants may be thinned out, to stand eighteen inches apart, and those plants that are taken up will do very well, transplanted in beds as above, giving them the same space. If the ground is well stirred, and the plants kept free from weeds while young, it will spread and be very luxuriant. As it stands the dry hot weather better than almost any other plant, it bears well till frost; as the leaves are plucked off for use, they will put out again.

SUMMER SAVORY

May be sown the last of March, or any time during the month of April, in small beds of almost any tolerable soil, drilled in rows nine inches apart, and covered lightly. Keep the ground loose, and free from weeds, during the growth of the plant.

SPRING TURNIP

May be sown the middle of February for early use, and again till the last of March for a succession, in any tolerably good, light soil, drilled in rows fifteen or eighteen inches apart, and covered one inch deep. As soon as the plants are well up, so as to be able to get hold of them with the fingers, thin them out to stand singly one or two inches apart; and as they advance in size, so as to crowd and touch each other, thin them out again so as to give them three or four inches space: afterwards they may be thinned out for use, giving them a little more space as they advance in size: keep the ground loose and light round the roots, and free from weeds. By this method the turnips will be always well rooted, and the tops very fine. Many persons have said, they never succeed in raising spring turnips, and for that reason have given up the cultivation of them. There are two very good reasons why these people are unsuccessful in their cultivation: one is, that they do not thin them out so as to give them sufficient space; and the next reason is, that they do not sufficiently work the ground, and keep them free from weeds. The author of this work has cultivated spring turnips for upwards of thirty years past, and has never failed one spring, when sown early, in having very fine large roots. The common late flat turnip may be sown from the first of August to the tenth of September, either in broadcast, or drilled in rows as the spring turnip, which would be preferable, in order to work or keep them free from weeds. They should have about eighteen or twenty inches space between the rows, or more, if the ground be strong. The large Norfolk field turnip should have two feet space between the rows, or more, if the ground be strong. New ground, enclosed a year before planting (where cows have used), is said to be preferable for fall turnips. Previous to sowing, plough it two ways, and run a harrow over it to level and break the ground loose. Hanover turnips may be sown from the twentieth of July to the middle of August: but the early sowing, the last of July or the first of August, will be best, if there should be a good season of rain, as the roots will then have time to get their growth before the winter sets in. They require a strong light soil, either spaded or well ploughed; they may be sown in drills twenty inches or two feet apart, and covered one inch deep. As soon as the plants will admit, thin them, to stand fifteen inches apart; those that are drawn out may be transplanted and do very well.

REMEDY FOR DESTROYING THE TURNIP-FLY.

Sir—I have been a turnip grower for the last twenty-five years, and, until 1815, to a considerable extent.

My remedy for destroying the turnip-fly is to get a quantity of lime from the kilns, in lumps or shells, which I put into a shed, or under cover, and slack it with tobacco water; when it is slacked into a powder I cause it to be sown carefully upon the young plants. If any farmer will try this simple remedy, his turnip crop may be saved from the destruction of the fly. Immediately after rain, or while the dew is on the turnip, is the best time for sowing the lime, when it adheres to the leaves of the young plants.

RUTA BAGA,

A late fall turnip, has a smooth leaf like a cabbage, and is known in the State of New York by the name of the yellow Russian turnip. There are other varieties similar, which have a leaf of a yellowish green, while the leaf of the ruta baga is of a bluish green, like the green of peas when nearly full grown, or like the green of a young and thrifty early York cabbage. The outside of the bulb of the ruta baga is of a greenish hue, mixed toward the top with a colour bordering on a red; and the inside of the bulb, if the sort be true and genuine, is of a deep yellow.

The time of sowing in the State of New York is from the twenty-fifth of June to the tenth of July; but as our seasons here are much longer, and the latter part of the summer generally hot and dry, it would be advisable not to sow sooner than the twentieth of July, and not later than the middle of August.

QUALITY OF LAND, MANNER OF SOWING, CULTIVATION, ETC.

As a fine rich garden mould, of a great depth, and having a porous stratum under it, is best for everything that vegetates, except plants that live best in water, so it is best for the ruta baga. But Cobbett, on the culture of this root, says: "There is no soil in which it may not be cultivated with great facility, except a pure sand, or very stiff clay." A few days previously to sowing, the ground must be ploughed up to a good depth into ridges, having two furrows on each side of the ridge, so that every ridge consists of four furrows, or turnings of the plough, making the tops of the ridges nearly or quite three feet from each other. As the ploughing should be deep, it will of course have a deep gutter between every two ridges. If the ground be not strong, rotten stubble manure may be placed under the middle of each ridge, beneath where the seed is sown. The ground being prepared, lay open a trench in each ridge or row, and sow the seeds very thinly, so that they may not touch each other, and cover them one inch deep, observing to press the ground well that the seeds may vegetate quickly before the earth gets too dry. This is always a good thing to be done even with any kind of seed that is sown lightly, especially in dry weather and under a hot sun. Seeds are very small things. When we see them covered over with the earth we conclude that all is safe, but if they do not vegetate and come up, they are then pronounced bad seeds; we should remember that a very small cavity is sufficient to keep them untouched nearly all around, in which case, under a hot sun, and near the surface, without they are well pressed after sowing, they are sure to perish. As soon as the plants are well up they may be thinned out so as to give them two or three inches space; and when the plants will admit they may be thinned out again, giving them fifteen inches space to stand. Those plants that are drawn out may be transplanted. As soon as the grass begins to make its appearance, the tops of the ridges around the plants may be hoed six inches in width. Then with a single horse plough take a furrow from the side of one ridge going up the field, a furrow from the other side coming down, then another furrow from the same side of the first ridge going up, and another from the same side of the other ridge coming down, observing to plough within three or four inches of the plant. This turns a ridge over the original gutter. Then observe to turn these furrows back again to the turnips. In this manner the weeds are nearly or quite all destroyed. When the weeds again make their appearance it will be necessary to repeat the same operation with the hoe and plough as before, which may suffice, unless the ground has been uncommonly grassy. Should it be necessary to work it the third time, the application of the hoe may answer. From the above mode of cultivation, the plants or leaves will be so productive as nearly to touch each other in the middle between the ridges. Cobbett states that from the above mode of cultivation, he has raised upward of a thousand bushels from one acre of ground on Long Island, New York, the turnips on an average weighing upward of seven pounds each. Transplanting is a mode said to be preferable, the ground ploughed up and made into ridges as above. The plants may be obtained either from those which are thinned out by the first mode of planting, or from seeds previously sown in small beds of a rich light soil, drilled in rows twelve inches apart. They should be thinned out as soon as they are well up, to stand two or three inches apart, in order that the plants may be more thrifty and regular in size. As soon as the plants are large enough, they may be transplanted, giving them the space above mentioned. A moderate season of rain is preferable to too much wet. The mode of planting is as follows: First, the hole is made sufficiently deep, deeper than the length of the root really requires; but the root should not be bent at the point, if it can be avoided; then, while one hand holds the plant with its root in the hole, the other hand applies the setting stick to the earth on one side of the hole, the stick being held in such a way as to form a sharp angle with the plant; then pushing the stick down so that its point goes a little deeper than the point of the root, and giving it a little twist, it presses the earth against the point or bottom of the root, and thus all is safe, and the plant is sure to grow. The general and almost universal fault is, that the planter, when he has put the root into the hole, draws the earth up against the upper part of the root or stem; and if he presses pretty well there, he thinks that the planting is well done: but it is the point of the root against which the earth ought to be pressed; for there the fibres are, and if they do not touch the earth closely, the plant will not thrive. The above mode will apply to cabbage and all other plants that are removed. If the ground was ploughed or prepared in the fall or winter before, so much the better (which should be done, as before observed,) only the ploughing should be very deep, and the ridges well laid up. In this situation it would, by the succession of frosts be shaken and broken fine as powder by March or April. It should then be turned back, always ploughing deep; then, previous to sowing, the manure may be put in the ridges and ploughed and sown as first described. As the winters at the North are too severe for the ruta baga, they are harvested or taken up the last of November, and either put in cellars or hills prepared in such a manner as to keep out the frost. In this climate they would keep in the ground during the winter without injury. The tops, as well as the roots, are excellent food for cattle, hogs or sheep. By cutting up the roots, and boiling or steaming them, with a little meal added, they are excellent food for sows and pigs.

STRAWBERRIES.

New beds of strawberries may be formed in this climate early in the month of September, made up in beds of four feet and a half or five feet wide, in a good light soil, neither too moist nor too dry. The most suitable manure for strawberries is composed of rotten leaves or decayed wood, mixed with other rotten vegetable substances scraped from the stable yard. Walks may be made between the beds, of about two and a half feet wide, sufficient to admit a wheelbarrow, for the purpose of manuring the beds from time to time as may be required. The plants may be procured from the roots that have formed from the runners on old beds, of the growth of the past season, or the year before, which would be preferable, as they would bear more abundantly the next season. Three rows may be set out in each bed, one row on each side, twelve inches from the border, and one row in the middle, so that the plants may have eighteen or twenty inches space from each other both ways: let them be covered two or three inches deep. Should the weather prove dry afterward they might occasionally be watered a few times of an evening, till they take root. Nothing more need be done, but keeping the soil light and loose between the plants, and free from weeds till frost. After the leaves have become dead or decayed, and before the ground freezes, they may be carefully taken off with the hand close to the crown of the root. The beds may then be covered two or three inches thick with a good coat of manure (half rotted) from the stable or cow-yard, or composed of decayed vegetable mould, as before stated, being careful that it be free from grass-seed of any kind. Early in the spring, before vegetation begins to grow, spread over the beds a slight covering of straw, and set fire to it: this will consume all the decayed leaves, &c., left from last season, and leave the whole neat and clean. The earth may be lightly turned in between the plants, being careful not to injure the roots; then spread on a thin coat of fine manure, well pulverized, raked from the yard, and mixed with ashes, which will warm the ground, and bring on the plants more speedily. After the plants are in a good growing state and begin to blossom, spread on a good covering of fine straw, two inches thick, when the straw is wet and the weather damp, taking care that it be spread on evenly, and that no part of the ground be left bare. This method brings on the fruit earlier, and ripens it finely, and produces a better quality: it likewise keeps the fruit clean, and free from dirt or sand. After this the vines should not be disturbed, until they have done bearing. As soon as the fruit is gone, the runners should occasionally be taken off as they appear, and the beds kept free from weeds during the summer, which may be done by hand as they show themselves. In the fall, when the leaves are decayed, the straw may be removed into the stable-yard, and mixed with other manure to rot. If any plants are then missing, they may be replaced with young plants, such as before stated. They should not be set later than the month of September. The beds may then have another coat or dressing, to preserve them from the severity of the winter, as before mentioned. If the above mode is adopted in the culture of the strawberry, they will bear and do well for many years.

NOTE.—Where they are male and female plants, such as the hautboys are stated to be, it would do well to mix the male plants regularly when setting out, in each row; say one male to every six female plants. The first row to commence with the first plant a male plant, and the second row to commence with the second plant a male plant, and the third row commencing with the third plant a male plant, and so on throughout the bed.

OBSERVATIONS ON THE CULTURE OF THE STRAWBERRY, BY A. J. DOWNING.

Botanic Garden and Nurseries, Newburgh, N. Y.

The strawberry is certainly one of the most valuable and delicious of all the smaller fruits. It is not easily cultivated. It yields an abundant crop in a short time, from a very limited space of ground; and while its pleasant sub-acid flavor is agreeable, and forms one of the most delightful additions to the dessert in summer, it is also extremely wholesome, never, as is the case with most other fruits, undergoing the acetous fermentation. In some diseases it has been highly beneficial, and it is affirmed that Linnæus was cured of the gout by an abundant use of the berries. The strawberry, though a low herbaceous plant, sends down remarkably strong roots. In good soils these are often found to penetrate to the depth of fifteen inches, or more, in a season. It is necessary, therefore, to produce a fine bed, that the soil be deep as well as rich : where the sub-soil is not positively bad the ground is always much improved by trenching (two spades deep) before setting the plants. In doing this, a good coat of manure should be deposited between the two spots. Old garden soils, which have been long cultivated, are astonishingly improved by this practice, the whole becoming renewed by the presence of the fresh soil ; and the growth of plants in such mould, when again acted upon by the sun and air, is of course proportionately vigorous. A deep yellow loam, rather damp than dry, is undoubtedly the preferable soil for this plant : but almost any soil, for so limited a species of culture, may, in the hands of a judicious gardener, be rendered suitable for it. We have seen splendid crops of fruit upon a very stiff, yellow clay, mellowed down by mixing with anthracite coal ashes and manure.

The best season for making new plantations of the strawberry is either in the spring, the latter part of February, or early in March, or directly after the beds have ceased bearing in August. If the latter time is chosen, the plants generally get sufficiently well established to bear a considerable crop the ensuing year. There are various modes in which to plant the beds when formed. Some arrange the plants so as to be kept in hills, others in rows, and others again allow them to cover the whole surface of the bed. We consider the first method preferable, as in that way the ground can be kept cultivated between the plants; the fruit is generally larger and finer, being more exposed to the genial influence of the sun, and the duration of the bed is greater. Three or four rows may be planted in each bed, at a suitable distance apart, and the runners from the rows should be shortened and cut off about three times during the season.

If the plants are not thriving well, a light top dressing between the rows in autumn will be of great advantage. Burning of the upper surface of the bed in the spring has been highly recommended by some persons; but we have never found it to answer our expectations upon trial. This fruit receives its name from the very ancient custom of placing straw on the beds between the rows of plants, to preserve the berries clean. Clean wheat or rye chaff may be substituted for straw, and it has the very great additional advantage of not only preventing most weeds from growing, by excluding the light, but also, by decomposing with considerable rapidity after the fruit season is past, it contributes much to the enrichment of the surface soil of the bed. Young and strong runners, well rooted, should in all cases be chosen to form the new bed, and not old plants, or those offsets which grow near them.

There is a fact with regard to the strawberry plant little known, the ignorance of which puzzles many a good cultivator. This is the existence of separate fertile and sterile or barren plants in many of the varieties, otherwise plants which produce chiefly male, and others that produce only female flowers. Botanically, the strawberry should produce both stamens and pistils in each flower, and the blossoms should consequently all mature fruit. This is really the case with the alpine, the wood strawberries, &c., but not entirely so with the large scarlet and pine strawberries. These latter sorts, it is well known, produce the largest and finest fruit, but we very often see whole beds of them in fine flowering condition, almost entirely unproductive. The common parlance in such cases is, that the variety has run out or degenerated; but the idea is a confused and ignorant one, while the healthy aspect of the plants fully proves the vigour of the sort. The truth is, in all strawberries of the foregoing classes, that although each blossom is furnished with stamens and pistils, yet in some plants the pistils are so few that they are scarcely perceived; in others there are scarcely any stamens visible. When the plants bear blossoms furnished with stamens only (or in a large proportion), they are, of course, barren; when pistils only are produced in abundance, they are fertile. To have a bed planted so as to bear abundantly, about one plant in eight or ten should be staminate, or barren blossoming plants, the others the fertile ones: for, if the latter only be kept, they alone will also be found unproductive. If any person will examine a bed of the Hudson, or any of the large scarlet strawberries, when they are in blossom, he will discover a great number of plants which bear large showy blossoms filled with fine yellow stamens. These are the barren plants. Here and there, also, he will discover plants bearing much smaller blossoms, filled with the heads of pistils, like a small green strawberry. The latter are the fertile ones. Now the vigour of the barren plant is so much greater than that of the fertile ones, and their offsets are so much more numerous, that if care be not taken to prevent this, they soon completely overrun and crowd out the fertile or bearing plants: and to this cause only is to be attributed the unproductive state of many beds of the large-fruited strawberries, which are in many instances perhaps entirely devoid of fertile plants.

The proper method, undoubtedly, is to select a few fertile plants of each kind, plant them in a small bed by themselves, and allow them to increase freely by runners; then, on planting, the proper proportion could be made, and kept up by the regular clipping of the runners.

Many of the fine English varieties of strawberries (Wilmot's superb, for instance) are generally found worthless here. This is owing, in some cases, to the ignorance or want of care of those persons who export the varieties, in sending often no fertile plants. In other instances it is equally owing to our negligence here, in not preserving the due proportion of barren and fertile plants. This peculiarity in the blossoms is very little known, or even understood, among scientific cultivators. It was first pointed out to us by our esteemed friend N. Longworth, Esq., of Cincinnati, one of our most distinguished western horticulturists. Its truth we have repeatedly verified, and a slight examination will convince any person of the cause of the numerous worthless yet thrifty looking strawberry beds throughout our gardens. The finest of the large English varieties of this fruit, which we cultivate here, is the Bishop. It is remarkably large, a most abundant bearer, and of superior flavor. Many of the larger-berried sorts, as the Methville Castle, have been hollow and comparatively tasteless, though of uncommon size. This variety, however, appears to us to unite all that can be desired to constitute a strong, fine, and delicious strawberry.

TOMATOES

May be sown any time in the month of April, in a light rich soil, drilled in rows four feet apart, where they are to remain and grow. They should be sown thinly, and covered one inch deep; and when the plants are well up, they may be thinned out three or four inches apart to give them a good regular growth. When they are several inches in height, thin them out again to stand three feet apart to remain; then put bushy sticks to them to bear them up, as they spread much and are inclined to run a little. By working them well, and keeping the ground loose and free from weeds, they will bear very abundantly till frost. After the tomatoes are once cultivated, people are not in the habit of saving the seed in the spring, but depend on the volunteer plants coming up from the rotten ones that decay and fall off on the ground in the fall; but to improve and have the genuine sort, it is best to select some of the largest and fairest for seed, and sow every spring. They should be squeezed out when fully ripe in water, rinsed well, and dried in the shade for several days. Spread them thinly before they are put away.

VINES.

Pumpkins may do well planted among corn, where the soil is very strong, and made light and loose; and in order that they may have room, it would be well to plant the corn in drills or rows six feet apart. The corn may be thinned out to stand two or two-and-a-half feet distance between each stalk, which mode is thought best for its growth. Between every other row the pumpkins may be planted, after the second ploughing and hoeing, in hills fifteen feet apart, making the hills nearly level with the ground. As the plants will admit, thin them out, so that only one vine may remain to a hill. Hoe and keep them free from weeds as long as it will admit without injury to the vines, observing not to hill up the earth around the root. Be sure to take off the first two or three crops when about as large as a goose egg. When the first crop of pumpkins is gathered, a larger number will occupy their place, which are to be trimmed off. The gathering may be continued so long as time is left for those on the vines to ripen. They are said to produce better planted apart from other vegetables. The ground should be strong, well pulverized, and made as level as possible, making the hills at least ten or twelve feet apart, keeping the ground loose and free from weeds, as in that mode of cultivation they are not likely to suffer from drought. They root at every joint, which makes it necessary to have the ground strong and kept loose as they run. All kinds of running squash may be planted about the first of April, and for a succession of crops may be planted till the middle of May, in a similar soil to the pumpkins. Plant free from other vegetables, and observe to take off the first growth when young, as with the pumpkins.

Summer-bush-squash for early use may be planted from the first to the twentieth of April, in a good, warm, light soil, in hills four feet apart. Put several seeds in a hill, but do not leave more than two or three good thrifty plants to grow in each, giving them ten or twelve inches space from each other. As they are cultivated, observe to draw the earth but lightly around the roots.

WINTER, OR LATE RUNNING SQUASHES.

The following method is recommended by a writer in the New England Farmer :—

A piece of ground not liable to suffer from drought, free from shade, and sheltered from wind, must be selected. At the proper season plough it three times, or till it is mellow. Dig holes in the earth at about eight feet distance. That will contain at least a bushel. Fill each hole about two-thirds full with good, strong, well rotted manure, and partly mixed with a good rotten compost taken from the hog-yard, or hog-pen, adding a pint of dry ashes or lime. Cover the manure slightly with some of the dirt first taken out of the hole, and, after a few days, work it all over thoroughly, and mix with it the best part of the dirt first thrown out, enough to fill up the hole, so as to be a little above the level of the ground. To allow for settling, repeat this working over two or three times in the course of ten or twelve days, and then plant seeds from good ripe squashes, which should be done about the last of April, or early in May. The plants will soon spring up and grow vigorously. The yellow-striped bug is the principal enemy to be dreaded. The plants, from the first appearance of the bug, should be examined twice a day, and the pest destroyed. Hoe the ground, and keep it loose and free from weeds, leaving not more than two thrifty plants to a hill. As the vines are liable to be blown about, it would be well to put brush between the hills for the tendrils to lay hold of as they spread. As the ground cannot be worked after the bushes are put down, and the vines spread, it should be kept very clean and free from weeds till then. The few weeds that come up after might be removed, or taken out with the hand.

DIRECTIONS FOR THE CULTIVATION OF WATER-MELONS.

From the Farmer's Register, Feb. 25, 1837.

Enclosed I send you a memorandum for the management of water-melons, by a gentleman who, in forty-three degrees of north latitude, frequently raises melons weighing from thirty to forty pounds. If the same pains were taken in the south, they might be raised very large and fine.

Dig holes two feet in diameter, twenty inches deep; fill one foot with rubbish raked from the garden and stable-yard, and unrotted manures; beat down hard, and water it freely; then fill to the top with rich soil; on this spread an inch of fine compost, or well rotted manure, compact but not hard. Plant the seed from the fifteenth of April to the first of May, ten or fifteen to a hill, to allow for accidents, a little below the surface of the compost. Brush over the hill with the hand so as to fill the holes made by the fingers; then cover the hill with an inch of clear sand. Should the weather be dry, water them well two or three evenings. The hills may be made twelve feet apart, and when the plants are well up they may be thinned out so as to leave five or six good thrifty plants: and when the plants have got six leaves thin out again, so that only two may remain to grow, and give the two plants ten or twelve inches space. If the season be dry, dig down by the side of the hills nearly as deep as the bottom of the holes, and put in a bucket or two of water, filling the hole after the water is absorbed. As soon as the yellow bug is gone, take away the sand, and supply its place with soil. This is all that can be done in the hill. When the plant has six leaves take off the centre shoot with the point of a sharp penknife, and when the lateral shoots are six inches long take off all but three. When these begin to fall to the ground, secure them down with cross sticks; and as they advance, spade up the ground a foot deep in advance of the vines. Once in every three or four feet, put a shovel full of soil on the leaf joint of the vine, not covering up the leaf, and press it down gently with the foot on both sides of the leaf. If this is kept moist, it will take root—the ends of the vines to be kept to the ground by cross-sticks. Let the vines spread from the hills regularly so as to cover the whole ground. If the side branches of the main vines are inclined to head up, and not to keep to the ground, take them off say a foot from the main vine. All pruning should be done in the middle of the day, when the sun shines. Let no melon set within four or five feet from the root, and then only one on a lateral branch, three to a plant. Let the vine run on as far as it will, keeping it to the ground. Permit no melon to grow that is deformed, and pull off no male blossoms.

When the melon has nearly attained to its size, others may be permitted to set on the same vine, and a second crop raised. I should think the vines might be made to grow from twenty to thirty feet long. Great care should be taken that the vines are not moved or trod upon.

Note.—The sand is put on the hills as a preventative against the yellow bug; but pumpkin or squash seed may be planted near the hills for the bugs to light on, taking care to pull them up as soon as the bugs are gone.

TO DRIVE BUGS FROM VINES.

The ravages of the yellow-striped bugs on cucumbers and melon vines, may be effectually prevented by sifting charcoal dust over the plants. If repeated two or three times the plants will be entirely free from annoyance. There is in charcoal some property so obnoxious to these troublesome insects, that they fly from it the instant it is applied.

HINT TO FARMERS.

It is said that the spirits of turpentine is a deadly enemy to all the insect tribes, and consequently will destroy the bug or worm which is found to prey on wheat and other grain. With a watering pot, finely perforated in the spout, a person may sprinkle a field of ten acres, without using more than two or three gallons. The experiment on a small scale may easily be tried.

TO CORRECT DAMAGED GRAIN.

Musty grain totally unfit for use, and which can scarcely be ground, may, it is said, be rendered perfectly sweet and sound by simply immersing it in boiling water, and letting it remain until the water becomes cold. The quantity of water must be double that of the grain to be purified. The musty quality rarely penetrates through the husk of the wheat; and in the very worst case it does not extend through the amylaceous matter which lies immediately under the skin. In the hot water all the decayed or rotten grain swims on the surface, so that the remaining wheat is effectually cleansed from all impurities without any material loss. It is afterwards to be dried on a kiln, occasionally stirring it, or it would dry in a hot sun if spread there. It should be effectually dried before it is ground, or there would be danger of its heating, and of the flour becoming musty.

A SUCCESSFUL MODE OF KEEPING SWEET POTATOES.

Dig a square pit in the ground about four feet deep, about the size you wish your house to be. Log it upon the inside until the logs are four or five feet above the surface of the earth. Draw the dirt well around the log frame. In the earth, on the inside of the first frame, build another frame of logs, leaving a space of one foot between the two. Fill the space between them with sand or dry earth. Upon the top of the frame lay a plank floor, the upper part of the floor to be covered with earth about four inches deep. Then a roof with the gable end opened at the south, and closed at the north. Have a door in the log frame about two feet square, to the south. After the potatoes are dug, they must be protected from the sides and bottom by dry pine leaves. The door must be kept open in warm dry days, and closed in cold damp weather, and always at night.

NOTE.—A floor of poles should be made to the potatoe house.

ANOTHER.

EDEN, EFFINGHAM Co., GA., May 16, 1843.

MR. EDITOR :—In your last number you invite communications upon the subject of preserving the sweet potatoe. As I have had some experience in that way, I will give you what I have found to be the most successful plan. Large hills or banks never keep so well as small ones; twenty bushels are sufficient. I open a hole or bed about a foot deep, in high dry land (deeper would be better) ; put the potatoes in a conical form, and cover with fine straw and corn stalks, or stalks alone, at first, and then with earth from eight to twelve inches deep ; covering lightly at first, and increasing the quantity of earth as the cold increases, would probably be better, but I have always found more risk in covering too lightly than too heavily. The only advantage in putting on stalks, is to keep the earth from mixing with the potatoes, as I have no doubt they would keep equally well, or better, to put the earth on without either straw or stalks. I built a house some years ago of clay, the walls about a foot thick, and covered (under the roof) in the same manner, but I found it would not preserve my potatoes. When I open a hill I now remove the contents to this house during winter; but in spring, say early in May, I remove my potatoes to a dry house or lot, for if left in the hill, they sprout or become too moist and soft to be good. I seldom keep the Spanish so late, but I rarely fail to have the yam till new potatoes are dug. C. POWERS.

PRESERVING IRISH POTATOES.

Injurious Effects of their Tops.

Everybody (except Cobbett, and he is dead) loves potatoes, that is, if, in the first place, they are ripe, in the second place well preserved, and, in the third place, they are well cooked. Without stopping to doubt the abilities of the good wives of our land in this department of household economy, we will proceed to read their husbands a homily upon the " ways and means" of preserving potatoes as they ought to be. We will suppose that they are ripe, that is, have obtained a fair size, and are mealy and farinaceous when properly cooked. When digging, do not let each boy or hand have a pile of his own, where he empties his basket, spreading them out as much as possible upon the ground, in order that each potatoe may feel the direct influence of the sun and air; and furthermore, do not let them dig more than can be got in at night, and therefore allowed to be out twelve or twenty-four hours with nothing over them but a few straggling tops, as a sort of apology for a covering. But if we may be allowed to advise in the premises—and we have followed plans, and by some spoiled as good potatoes as ever were grown by our ignorance or carelessness, or both—we recommend a cart, covered on the top tightly with boards, or by an old coverlid, so that the potatoes when put in shall not be exposed at all to the light, and as little possible to the air, and carried into the cellar or bins as soon after they are taken from the hills as they can be conveniently. The bins should also be so constructed that potatoes can be excluded from air and light—in short, so as to keep them in a state similar to that which they are in previously to their being dug, that is, secure from the light and air, with a little moisture and a temperature sufficiently low to keep them from vegetating.

The plan laid down by Mr. Barnum, and published in our paper last summer, we think is a good one, viz., to make a bin. Put some sand or turf at the bottom, cut some sods and line up the ends with them, and when the potatoes are put in, cover them over with sods, and beat them down solid. This keeps them moist and cool, and, we doubt not, is an excellent plan. The light has a peculiar action on some potatoes, making them heavy and watery or waxy, and strong or rancid to the taste. It is, perhaps, not always possible to prevent this when they have suffered from some disease of their tops, or have been disturbed while growing, or have not a suitable soil. As it regards the tops, it is generally the custom to throw them down, and take no further trouble about them. A correspondent in a late number of the Farmer recommends preserving them when they are green for fodder; and another correspondent cautions us against leaving them on the ground, because they form a harbor and breeding-place for insects, which will injure the next crop, especially if it be wheat. We know not whether this invariably follows; but we have seen during the past summer several crops of wheat that succeeded a potatoe crop, all of which were injured by some worm or insect. One, in particular, we recollect in the neighborhood of our office, a part of which was much injured and very thin,— while another end of the same field, and on soil of the same texture, but which had not been preceded by potatoes, was very stout and prolific. It is better, therefore, undoubtedly, either to gather them up and burn them, or throw them into the hog-yard, for their shoatships to manufacture into manure.—*Me. Farmer.*

ANOTHER MODE OF PRESERVING POTATOES FOR FOOD.

An English paper says that to preserve potatoes in a proper state for food for many years, it is only necessary to scald them, or subject them to a heated oven for a few minutes. By doing this they will never sprout, and the farinaceous substance will keep good for many years, provided the cortical part or skin be entire. They should be well dried after being scalded.

TO IMPROVE THE QUALITY OF THE IRISH POTATOE.

MOORFIELD, Feb. 18, 1821.

MR. SKINNER,—I had heard, many years back, that the best way to improve the potatoe was from the seed of its own apple. About five or six years past I made the trial. I gathered a handful of the apples of the blue potatoe when fully ripe. I washed them, and washed out the seed, and dried them. In the spring I sowed them in drills. They came up very thick, having the appearance of small weeds. In two or three weeks they put out leaves, having the appearance of potatoes. I then thinned and worked them as I thought right. In the fall I had seeds of many kinds, white, blue, and red, of various shapes and complexions. I selected four or five kinds in the spring, and planted each separately, and found I had improved my potatoes very much as to the flavor, and also some of the kinds I had selected were very productive, so much so that I planted no more of my old seed, and do still consider the change advantageous.

ABEL SEYMOUR.

ON THE CULTURE OF THE GRAPE VINE.

From the Journal of the American Silk Society.

There are few things that afford more pleasure for the expense of time and trouble, than a good and well managed grape vine. From considerable observation, the editor of this Journal was led to conclude, that a very erroneous practice was generally pursued in relation to grape vines; and three years ago, determined to try an experiment. The error in practice alluded to, is this: the vine is permitted to grow to the full extent of its ability, and thus every season a large portion of wood has to be cut off, and thrown away. It occurred to the writer, that this waste of the power of the plant, might, and ought to be prevented. Accordingly in the spring of 1837, he obtained an Isabella vine, one year old from the layer, having a very good root, and planted it in an ordinary soil, of rather a sandy quality, putting a wheelbarrow load of woodyard manure and old lime mortar about the root. As soon as it began to grow, he rubbed off all the buds but one, and trained that perpendicularly, rubbing off during the season all side shoots; and when it had reached to the top of a second story balcony, nipped the end off, thus stopping its further growth. In the spring of 1838, he rubbed off every bud but two at the top of the vine, and trained these two along the front of the balcony, having stretched a large wire along the posts for their support. He rubbed off every side bud, during the season, as at first. Both shoots made about thirty-five feet of growth this season. In the spring of 1839, every joint on the horizontal shoots was permitted to send forth its buds, and to grow unmolested, till the branches had fairly set fruit, generally until they were about eighteen inches long. Then the end of each branch was nipped off, and its further growth prevented. The perpendicular stem was carefully prevented from sending out buds. The whole plant was carefully watched that no more buds might be permitted to grow—each one being rubbed off as soon as it appeared. Thus from about the middle of June, the vine was not permitted to form any new wood. During the season the grapes grew uncommonly well, and every one ripened in good season, and was very fine, as was proved by the numerous company at the Horticultural Society exhibition, who unanimously pronounced them the finest grapes there. The produce of the vine was three hundred and fifteen bunches, all very large, and the berries of uncommon size. The society awarded to them its first premium for native grapes. Almost everybody, however, doubted whether the plant had not been injured by this excessive bearing of fruit; and many old gardeners considered that it would be killed by it. The writer never doubted on this score. He had only compelled the plant to make fruit, instead of wood, to be cut off and thrown away; and has no doubt that if he had been able to get the season before a greater length of wood for fruit branches, the plant would have supported a much larger quantity of fruit. On trimming the vine preparatory to its bearing in 1840, there was very little wood to be cut off. Only two buds were left on each branch of last year's growth, and these are now growing, and showing fruit buds very finely. The vine is not dead, nor does it appear to have been injured in the least by last year's hard work. So far, the experiment is beautifully successful, and we now feel authorized to recommend this plan to all who love fine fruit. It must be borne in mind that the experiment was made with the Isabella grape; we of course cannot say anything about its applicability to other kinds from experience; but the same reasoning applies with equal force to all kinds. If the powers of a plant can be turned from the formation of wood, to that of making fruit, as we have proved it can be, in the case of the Isabella grape, we do not see any reason why the experiment may not be successful with all kinds of grapes and fruit. One thing we do know, that a plant that bears fruit does not grow as much as one that does not; and we are hence authorized to infer, that the power of the plant may be directed at pleasure, either to the growth of fruit or of wood—that by suppressing the one, you may increase the other, to a very great extent. The vine above described has attracted the attention of numerous persons, and many have determined to follow the example. It may be observed that this vine occupies no room at all in the garden. It grows close in the corner of the house, a single stem ascending fourteen feet to the balcony, when it starts off horizontally as above described, along the balcony. Thus every house in any city that has a yard at all, so that the vine may be set in the earth, may have just such a supply of delicious grapes as the writer of this had last fall. G. B. S.

ANOTHER MODE ON THE CULTURE OF THE VINE.

Why vineyards should have so little attention bestowed upon them now, when there are many thousands of acres of poor land in our country that are of little value in any agricultural point of view, but on which vines would flourish and produce largely, and yield a profitable return, is truly surprising. The present mode of culture offers ample means for procuring an abundant supply of this delicious fruit, for hundreds of pounds might annually be produced upon the surface of walling; for every house in town and country has more or less spare walling, which is deemed of no value, and might be turned into invaluable account in the production of the fruit of the vine. There is not a single point of culture in the whole routine of the management of the vine, the knowledge of which is so important as that which enables the cultivator to discover with accuracy the greatest quantity of fruit he can annually extract from it without checking its growth, or impairing its vital powers; for it is well known, that the generous flavor of grapes, and the vital energies of the vine, are much affected by over cropping. No vine under three inches in girth ought to be suffered to ripen any fruit, and the great end to be attained is the flavor of the grape that is used for the table, and this is regulated by the circumstances under which they ripen; one of which is, the quantity of grapes suffered to remain and ripen as compared with the strength of the vine. Some vines show more fruit than others, but the power to ripen is nearly equal in all. The warmer the aspect, the greater perfection does the grape attain in our climate, as is already demonstrated in the hothouses of our distinguished fellow-citizen, N. Biddle, Esq.; but it is not warmth alone, shelter is equally necessary. There is no period in the growth of the vine, from the moment it is planted until it attains the greatest extremity of its growth, in which any movement of the wind will not have a greater or less pernicious effect on its well-being; for its perspiration is so great through its large leaves, that a great supply of fat is necessary every moment through the growing season to enable it to recruit its loss. Every wind that blows on the foliage of the vine deranges its functions, and retards the growth of the plant, and the ripening of its fruit, in proportion to its duration and violence. An aspect due south is a very good one, but the southwest winds form a drawback to its excellence. The best is east by north; tolerably good grapes may thus be grown. I have seen the black Hamburgh attain great perfection in this aspect. The soil most congenial to the growth of the vine is a light rich sandy loam. One reason why grapes will not ripen on open walls is, the great depth of mould in which the roots of vines are suffered to run, which supplies them with too great a quantity of moisture. The subsoil should be of dry materials, for it is not mere earth the roots require, but air also; and every root wants a peculiar temperature in which they thrive best, and they flourish better in a stony soil than any other.

ANOTHER.

The suggestions below, as to the use of lime around fruit trees, are worthy of attention. In the autumn of 1841, we laid bare the roots of a number of unthrifty apples, pear, and peach trees, and left them exposed during the winter, returned the dirt in the spring, and applied to the roots of each tree about half a bushel of gas lime. Last year the trees seemed greatly improved, and the pears bore more than three times as much as they did the two previous years; the limbs had to be propped up, and the fruit seemed improved. We treated some old quince trees in a similar manner; and the influence was obviously beneficial. Ashes are a good substitute for lime, and ordinary lime would probably do as well as the gas lime. Exposing the roots of trees occasionally during the winter, it is well known, is very beneficial.

Nov. 22, 1842.

I have perfect faith in the beneficial use of calcareous substances applied to the roots of trees, sensible, as one of your correspondents has observed, that "oxygen is the basis of acidity," with which all putrid substances are charged; and it is with this view that Major Reybold, of Delaware, the first of the culvators of the peach (for he and his sons, and sons-in-law, now number 70,000 peach trees planted in orchards), is at this time actively engaged in dressing his trees with shell-marl by depositing a quantity at the root of every tree, to be pulverized by the frosts of the ensuing winter. He also cultivates his orchard with the plough, turning a shallow furrow over the whole surface of the land, three times during the summer,—a weighty affair, seeing that one of these orchards contains more than one hundred acres; by these means he conceives that he renovates the land and benefits the health of the trees, which are indeed in full vigor, although many of them are very old, and the size of some apple trees of mature growth. I remember also, that Mr. Dager, one of the proprietors of the lime quarry, mentioned at page 309 of the fourth volume of the Cabinet, the lime from which was proved by analysis to yield 96. 6 per cent. of carbonate, and not a trace of magnesia, increased the size of the fruit of an apricot tree three fold, by digging in around its roots a quantity of lime, adding also to its flavor in an equal degree.

Peach Worm.—L. Physic, of Philadelphia, says a mixture of one ounce saltpetre, and seven ounces salt, applied on the surface of the ground, in contact and around the trunk of a peach tree, seven years old and upwards, will destroy the worm, prevent the yellows, and add much to the product and quality of the fruit. He also sows the orchard with the same mixture, at the rate of two bushels to the acre.

MANAGEMENT OF FRUIT TREES.

Messrs Editors,—The article in the June number of the present volume of your paper, headed the Peach Tree, requires some notice, and probably a much more extended one than my time will admit at present. In the first place, allow me to say that the disease of the peach tree called and known as the yellows, is not contagious, and I will hold myself ready to prove, not theoretically or speculatively, but practically, that there is no such thing as a healthy peach tree being infected by another standing adjacent and having the yellows. I will not say that this or any other disease cannot be inoculated ; but if it can, I have not been able to do it in several experiments made for the purpose.

I will endeavor to detail some of my experiments and observations in regard to the yellows, &c., and believe that I can show it to be the result of error in their culture. This farm had upon it in 1836, a small apple orchard, the trees standing at distances of thirty-two feet; between the rows of apple trees, peach trees were planted, at distances of sixteen feet tree from tree. The peach trees were in a very unhealthy condition; some of them, being in the last stage of the disease called the yellows, ceased to live after that year; others not so bad, but having the disease in the worst form (every part of the tree being affected), received my care and attention. My first desire was to get rid of the peach worm, which I readily accomplished by the use of salt and saltpetre around the trunks of the trees, &c., and at the same time I gave to those trees producing good fruit, a top dressing of manure. In 1838-39, my orchard was entirely free from the worm, and appeared in a healthy condition, with the loss of only three trees out of about forty that had the yellows.

The orchard being in good health, I resolved to test my then theoretical views; having planted a few trees to supply me with fruit in case these should be destroyed, I went more cheerfully to work, and selected eight trees standing in a row, and had the ground manured for about ten or twelve feet on each side of the row of trees; it was then ploughed and potatoes were planted in every third furrow, this furrow receiving an additional quantity of manure. The balance of the orchard was ploughed during the month of September; a part thereof received a dressing of manure and was ploughed in; another part was, manured after being ploughed, and a third part without manure; the whole orchard was sown with wheat, and the following spring with clover. The effect was, that a large majority of the peach trees showed some symptoms of disease, but more perceptible on those where there was no manure, where the manure was turned under, and where the potatoes were planted. Of the eight trees where the potatoes were planted, I was resolved on saving four of them if possible, for here I thought the greatest amount of injury was done (though I have thought differently on this subject since), yet in this case the injury met my fullest expectation, and the four trees unattended to had the yellows and were about to die, when Mr. J. L. M'Knight and a friend of his, both living in or near Bordentown, N. J., and both peach growers, came to see my orchard; these gentlemen, pointing to three of these trees, asked if I could cure them; I told them it might be possible, but they were very far gone; their remark was, that they thought these trees could not be restored to health. The middle one of these three trees, being most diseased, was selected by me to be cured; and if Mr. M'Knight and his friend will call and see me in September next, I will promise to give them some perfectly sound fruit, to be gathered from this tree, though the fruit is not of a very good kind. The other two trees died for want of attention, and were cut down this spring. Now this is one instance of which I have ample testimony of this disease being curable, though it is not the first instance of cure with me by very many. The disease was produced by the plough, and the cure by rest, with a top dressing of stable manure and ashes.

I deem it unnecessary to say anything more about my orchard at present, but beg your indulgence to permit me to ask attention to the effect produced from ploughing orchards. A person living within two miles of me, has an apple orchard that was, to within the last three years, a most prolific orchard, but in consequence of some of the trees putting on the appearance of decay, he though that to manure it and plough it would be of service; this he did three years ago, and the orchard producing no fruit the next year, and the trees appearing more unhealthy, he manured and ploughed again; but still he has no fruit, and his trees are growing worse instead of better. Another person about seven miles distant, has an apple orchard that he has worked in corn three years ago; one of his people being at my house the year following, I enquired if there was any fruit on the trees: " No! the frost has killed all the apples." I then asked him about trees standing in different parts of the orchard, where I know they could not plough, and was told these trees were full of fruit, and that the " frost did not hurt them." I desired him to say, the next time he was asked why these trees were full of fruit and the others, that they could not injure them with the plough barren. I could give very many instances of this kind, but my object being to call attention to this matter, I will ask every one to make his own observations and comparisons; let every farmer look into his neighbor's orchard and his own, and see what the effect of ploughing is when compared with the unploughed orchard adjacent to that ploughed; let him call to recollection the fine orchard planted by his father, that is going into decay, and ask himself the cause, and he will receive more knowledge upon this subject than could be derived from volumes written upon orchards—though I would strongly recommend the perusal of all works written upon the subject of our business; the avocations of life are always promoted by a proper and strict inquiry after truth, and no agent should be neglected to the advancement of so desirable an end.

My system is to work a tree just as I do the corn plant; the one as an annual, the other as a perennial; give the tree all the cultivation it is to have while young, and before a set of organs are wanted for the perdurable formation of fruit; and when the tree puts on the appearance of premature decay, I give it a coat of manure spread upon the surface of the ground: this I apply in the fall of the year, always preferring long to short manure, and when ashes are deemed necessary, I have put them on in the spring.

Shall I say a word here about peach trees 30 or 40 years ago, which Mr. Downing represents to have grown anywhere in the United States, south of 43° of latitude? Well, 40 years ago there was but little demand for peaches as a market fruit, and they were for the most part converted into pork and brandy. For these purposes, it did not answer at that period of time, to pick them off the trees by hand, but a neat grass lay was considered as indispensable to facilitate their collection, as step-ladders are at the present day. The peaches then were shook off the trees, and the best selected, either for drying or for the still, and the hogs disposed of the balance.

There were several reasons why orchards were not destroyed at that time by tillage, and perhaps the most prominent one was that a grain crop in the orchard would prevent or retard the gathering of the peaches, which, by the by, were worth more than any grain crop that could be grown in the orchard; but whenever an old peach orchard was ploughed a few times, a new one had to be planted, or at least such was the case 30 years ago, on some farms, to my certain knowledge. I do not wish to be understood that the peach tree can be grown at the present time with the same facility it could then, for I have no doubt that the pabulum necessary for the support of this tree has become in a great measure exhausted from the soil, but I presume it can be restored; if so, we must get "the neighbors" to resuscitate their soils and to form a good stock by proper tillage; but when the trees come into full bearing, we must then feel satisfied with whatever Nature may be pleased to do in the premises, for any stirring of the soil after this period of growth is obtained, has a tendency to bring the orchard into decay, of which I can show hundreds of surviving witnesses.

A careful inquiry will show that the peach tree began to decline about the close of our last war with England; grain commanding a very high price at that time, peaches were only considered in a secondary point of view, and orchards that probably had not been disturbed with the plough for 15 or 20 years previous, were then put in wheat, corn, &c. This soon brought the orchards into decay, and in many instances they were not replaced; and when replanted, they have been treated very differently from the original. We must now have a crop of grain, grass, or roots, but in former times such things were not expected from a peach orchard after it began to produce full crops of fruit.   LITTLETON PHYSICK.

Ararat Farm, Md., June 28, 1843.

TO PRUNE GRAPE VINES TO ADVANTAGE.

In pruning vines leave some new branches every year, and take away (if too many) some of the old, which may be of great advantage to the tree, and will much increase the quantity of fruit. When you train your vine leave two knots or buds, and cut them off the next time; for usually the two buds yield a bunch of grapes. Vines when thus pruned have been known to bear abundantly, whereas others that have been cut close, to please the eye, have been almost barren of fruit.

REMEDY AGAINST MILDEW OF GRAPES.

Take a pint and a half of sulphur, and a lump of the best unslacked lime of the size of the first; put these in a vessel of about seven gallons measurement: let the sulphur be thrown in first, and the lime over it; then pour in a pailful of boiling water, stir it well, and let it stand half an hour: then fill the vessel with cold water, and after stirring well again, allow the whole to settle. After it has become settled, dip out the clear liquid into a barrel, and fill the barrel with cold water, and it is then fit for use. You next proceed with a syringe holding about a pint and a half, throwing the liquid with it on the vines in every direction, so as completely to cover the foliage, fruit, and wood. This should be particularly done when the fruit is just forming and about one-third the size of a pea, and may be continued twice or thrice a week for two or three weeks. The whole process for one or two hundred grape vines need not exceed half an hour.

ON THE CULTURE OF THE PEACH TREE.

[Published by order of the Agricultural Society of Fayette County]

The subscriber having bestowed much of his time

and attention on the cultivation and preservation of fruit trees, and willing to diffuse any knowledge he may possess on the subject, submits, for the benefit of the public at large, the following results of many experiments. He has found, after adopting various modes in rearing the peach tree, that none succeeds so well as the following: In the fall of the year I bury the peach stones (from which I design to raise trees) in a hole under six or eight inches of earth, to remain there until the following spring, when I take them up, and after cracking the stone carefully, so as not to injure the kernels (most of which will be found swollen and ready to sprout), I then plant them in a trench eight or ten inches apart, where they are suffered to remain until the plant has acquired a growth of three or four inches in height, when I transplant them to the place designed for my peach orchard, placing small stones about the plant, to preserve them from being trod upon by the cattle, &c. It is unnecessary to be more explicit on this part of the subject; every farmer is acquainted with the mode of rearing, which is emphatically trifling, compared with the preserving of this valuable and delicious fruit tree. Few have turned their attention to it, and of the few the smallest number have succeeded: perhaps none have succeeded fully in preserving the peach tree from decay for any length of time. I have, however, prevented the destruction of my trees for several successive seasons, and am entirely convinced of the efficacy of my plan in destroying an insect, which, of all other things, I believe most pernicious to the tree. It is a fact, of which perhaps few farmers are aware, that the peach tree receives its death by an insect of the fly kind, which annually deposits its eggs in the bark of the root of the tree, sometimes at or near the surface of the ground, but most generally under the surface. The egg is deposited by making small perforations : these are sometimes numerous, and from the circumstance of a gum issuing out of the wounded parts, there is no doubt but that it materially injures the health of the tree. Knowing this to be a fact, and believing the insect just alluded to, to be the primary, if not the sole cause of the failure of our peach orchards, I tried a variety of methods to destroy them, and found the following to have the desired effect : In the fall of the year (at which time the eggs are deposited) I take for a grown tree a handful of tobacco stems, or what will do equally as well, about half a gallon of wood ashes; and after baring the roots, lay either of them on and about the trunk, and cover the whole with earth. The amber of the tobacco, and the ley of the ashes, are both fatal to the embryo insect, and will effectually destroy it. For young and healthful trees a much smaller quantity will do, as they are seldom disturbed by the insect, from the circumstance of their roots being less exposed than those of an old tree.

Many farmers, in my opinion, injure the health of peach trees, and bring on premature decay by pruning. I have tried them with and without pruning, and am decidedly against using the pruning hook at all. The reasons in favor of this plan are obvious. I suffer the tree to grow as Nature pleases, which it does in the manner best calculated to withstand the shocks of storms, and to bear its fruit without props. In pursuing an opposite plan, by cutting off the first branches that appear, a long body is formed, and the tree ultimately divides in two or three main branches, which, when loaded with fruit, or during high winds, are apt to split asunder, and the death of the tree ensues. It is true I have found it necessary sometimes to prop my trees; but they never attain a great height, and take the shape which is given to them by nature. The load is so equally distributed that the necessary propping is easily done. In addition to what I have already stated, it may not be improper to add, that an intelligent farmer informed me, that merely to keep the earth about the root of the tree in the fall of the year, and removing it again when the winter sets in, would destroy the insect, whose eggs would then be exposed to the severe frost. I have never tried this experiment, but am of opinion that it would have a good effect. It is from its simplicity well worthy a trial.

Note.—I prefer ashes, because they are always at hand, and because they are really a good manure for peach trees. I have found a sandy soil best, both for a nursery and orchard. John Hackney.

PLANTING APPLE ORCHARDS.

Communicated.

The following mode of planting an orchard of apple trees is possessed of many advantages over the old method. According to the common mode, the trees are planted at fifty feet every way, both to give them room to grow, and spread to their full extent, and to work the ground between them for their benefit, and the crop produced. The disadvantages arising from this plan are so many, so great, and so fatal, as to have suggested the one now proposed in place of it.

The disadvantages attending the usual mode of cultivation are,

1st. The trees grow up with a straight body, six or seven feet high, before they are suffered to produce their limbs. This large body is soon filled with worms under the bark, which is pecked into holes all around by the small woodpecker searching after them. These two causes soon bring on the canker, which in a little time causes the decay and death of the trees.

2d. They frequently grow crooked and deformed, which is not only unsightly but a great injury.

3d. Their bodies and large branches become full of moss, and harbor insects which prey upon them.

4th. The trees planted thus, and especially where the ground is cultivated between them, grow luxuriantly, throw out large branches, and form high trees with great heads: thus exposing them to the fury of the winds, which sometimes break off large branches, and which, whenever it happens, if care (which is very seldom given) is not taken to smoothe the wound, and protect it from the air, bring on disease and decay. It also renders the fruit liable to be blown down, to the great loss of the proprietor. They are, besides, more difficult to prune and keep in order. Their fruit is more difficult and expensive to gather, owing to the height and extent of the head, and they seldom bear more than every other, or every third year.

By the mode below suggested all these disadvantages, it is believed, will be avoided. The trees are to be planted at every twenty feet; the second spring after planting, head them down at about three feet from the ground, so as to let four branches arise from the part left, taking care to pare away the part from the highest branch down close, so as to let the growing bark cover the wound as soon as possible. This ought always to be well covered with Forsyth's composition, until the scar is completely overgrown by the new wood. The following spring prune all the four branches, which ought to be trained as regularly as they can be had on all sides of the body, each about a foot long, and suffer each of them to put out two shoots, rubbing off with the finger all beside them. Thus you will have from this time eight branches to form its head, and a body only about two feet long. All these eight branches are to be suffered to grow until the tree comes into bearing, taking care to suffer no strong growing spongy shoot to grow beyond its fellows, but keeping all of equal growth and size. When the tree comes to bear, four of these branches, each alternate one all around the tree, is to be headed down, each to its lowest shoot, which is to be trained in the vacancy of its parent branch, which has been lopped away. While these four branches are in the progress of making new wood, the four that have been left are bearing, which they will do in plenty for three, four, or five years, until the new wood has come into a bearing state, which may be known by the fruit buds which they will show in plenty in every part. When these new branches have arrived at this state, then cut out the four old ones that have borne fruit, and are now getting up pretty high, and bearing mostly on their tops. Take care in cutting out these old branches to do it as low as you can, and where their lowest shoot is, however small, or where there is even the appearance of a bud to shoot forth and renew them. These are to be trained in the same manner as before directed for the first that were cut out, until they arrive at the state and size to bear fruit in their turn again, when the last bearing ones once more undergo the same operation, and so on alternately. A tree cultivated in this manner may bear for a hundred, or it may be two hundred years.

Note particularly in pruning, or in cutting away these branches, that it must be always done so near to the shoot or bud that grows to furnish the branch in the place of the one cut away, that the growing wood may cover the wound as soon as possible. In all cases where the knife is used, or any injury done in any way, the part must be smoothed, and the composition applied without delay, at any season. The stems, or bodies of the trees, and the branches, are once a year at least to be washed with soft soap and water, which, by encouraging their growth, and preventing moss and insects from harboring therein, is of essential service to them. The advantages of this mode are,

1st. The bodies being so short are easily kept clear and free from insects, and of course from the wounds made by the wood-pecker in searching for them, and thus kept healthy and thriving, and of course highly fruitful.

2d. They cannot but be straight, with as many branches on the one side as the other, by which the sap is regularly dispersed, conducing to the beauty, regularity, and health of the trees.

3d. The trees are thus kept in perpetual youth, health, and fertility, and yield an annual crop.

4th. They are not subject to be broken by the high winds, nor their fruit to be lost by being broken off.

5th. They can never contract moss on either body or branches, which greatly injures the large tree.

6th. Their fruit is easily thinned, and more easily gathered, and at less expense; and lastly, the pleasure arising from an orchard thus growing and thus kept would be much greater, and of course procure for it more care and attention.

Let any one go through the State, or the United States, and I will venture to say, that he will find almost every orchard with the body of the trees drilled in holes, and their branches covered with moss, many of the trees bent and crooked; much old, naked, barren, and even dead wood upon them, and scarcely one that bears every year. To all those whose orchards are in this state, this mode offers the only way to resuscitate and renovate them. Cut down any that are crooked, wounded, irregular, diseased, or decayed, and train up the best and strongest shoot that will put up from the part left, or from the root, and by managing them as above directed, in a few years a young, healthful orchard, will take the place of an old, cankery, decayed, unsightly, unfruitful, and unproductive one. It is scarcely necessary to add, that the more the ground is stirred between the trees the more they will grow and flourish. The best manure for them is marsh mud; salt marsh, if to be had, but never fresh stable manure. The salt in the mud conduces to the health of the trees, destroys slugs, worms, and insects, and this manure carries no weeds into the orchard.

A comparison of the productiveness and profit of an orchard cultivated in the old way, with one treated in the manner now proposed, will show the superiority of the latter over the former in a strong point of view. An acre will contain only sixteen trees at fifty feet apart, whereas it will contain two hundred at twenty feet; the first only bears every other year. Let us then take them when come into full bearing, and see their product for a space of ten years. We will allow each large tree to bear twenty bushels; this will give 16 by 20=320 bushels for the acre; and as the trees only bear half the time, consequently in the ten years they will produce sixteen hundred bushels. Allow only five bushels per tree for the small orchard, the hundred trees in the acre will produce five hundred bushels, and as they bear every year, the ten years will give five thousand bushels. If it be said the allowance of five bushels is too much for a small tree, let the objector remember that this tree is always in a healthy and fruitful state; that its bearing being renewed every four or five years, it is always young and lusty, and able to bear a good crop. Let it also be remembered that an average of twenty bushels to the large trees is a great allowance, which I will venture to say is never realized. Thus, then, whether we consider the beauty, the regularity, the health, or the vigor of the trees on the plan proposed; their greater fruitfulness, and consequent profit; their perpetual renovation and youth; the ease with which their superabundant fruit is thinned and gathered; their greater exemption from injuries from high winds; we cannot but perceive that the advantages are so many, and so decisive, as to give the plan a marked superiority. With best wishes for the continued usefulness of your well conducted paper, to the great interest of the country, I contribute my mite.

RUSTICUS.

FRUIT TREES.

The new method of raising fruit trees by planting the scions is a great desideratum in the art of obtaining good fruit. It has many advantages over grafting, because it is more expeditious, and requires no stock or tree. They may be planted where they are required to stand, and the labor for one day will be sufficient to plant out enough for a large orchard. After the scions are obtained, the method of preparing the plant is as follows: Take the scion as for grafting, and at any time after the first of February, and until the buds begin to grow considerably, and dip each end of the shoot in melted pitch, wax, or tallow, and bury it in the ground, the buds uppermost, while the body lies in a horizontal position, and at the depth of two or three inches. We are informed that trees obtained in this way will bear in three or four years from the time of planting. We have no doubt of the practicability of this method of raising fruit.

A gentleman in this vicinity the last season planted about twenty scions of different kinds of pears, which appear to flourish. The composition he used was melted shoemaker's wax.—*Cultivator*.

PLUGGING TREES.
From the Evening Post.

This operation is a very efficient remedy for destroying caterpillars, and other insects, preying upon the limbs of fruit trees, &c.

It has often been desired to find such a remedy. Our shade trees are covered every year with disgusting and voracious caterpillars. Year after year, new, troublesome, and costly means are proposed, which are inefficient; while this very easy and cheap way to poison and destroy at once all the insects of any tree is so little known, that our farmers and gardeners appear to be unacquainted with it. It was discovered in France, and I have verified it by the knowledge of it everywhere. This simple operation consists in boring a hole with a large spike gimblet about one third the diameter of the tree in depth. Fill the hole nearly full with the flour of sulphur, and plug it up by driving in a wooden peg. This does not injure the tree in the least, but the sulphur is decomposed, or carried into the circulation by the sap, and is exhaled by the leaves in a gaseous state, while it poisons and kills all the caterpillars and insects preying upon them. C. S. RAFINESQUE, *Prof. of Botany.*

THE CANKER WORM.
From the Farmers' Gazette.

Take one gallon of cheap whale oil, one pound flour sulphur, twelve ounces sal ammoniac, and one pound chloride of lime. Let the sal ammoniac and lime be made fine, so that all parts may mix together. Take some old or cheap woollen cloth (about nine inches wide, and in length according to the size of the tree), and tie it round about the middle so as to encircle the tree, letting the upper part of the cloth hang over like the collar of a coat, so as to form a curve for the millers to run into. The cloth may be dipped in the mixture, or it may be well to spread it on with a paint brush, and it may be well to renew it once or twice a week till the millers have done flying. This was tried last season, after the worms were fully grown. Being shaken from the trees, t ey attempted to ascend, and would die in two minutes after they came in contant with the above ingredients. DAVID RITNER.

New Haven, Jan'y 27th, 1841.

ANOTHER.—" Capt. Chancey Treat, of East Hartford, has discovered a complete remedy against the ravages of the canker-worm, simply encircling the tree at the surface of the ground with Scotch snuff. The writer of this has examined the trees on Capt. Treat's premises, and found the circle of snuff completely fringed with thousands of dead worms. These trees were all tarred, and where the snuff was used, no worms appeared on the tar, and where the snuff was omitted the insects nearly covered the tar."

COMPOSITION FOR HEALING WOUNDS IN TREES.

Melt a pound of tar with four ounces of tallow, and half an ounce of saltpetre, and stir the whole together. A coat of this composition, applied to a cut or bruise, will prevent its decay, and cause the wound to heal. Before applying it, all unsound timber should be cleared away.—*Hartford Courant.*

CEMENT FOR GRAFTING.

Two pounds and two ounces of resin, six ounces of tallow, and ten ounces of beeswax. Melt them together, and turn the mixture into cold water, and let it remain till cool enough to handle; then work it as shoemakers' wax. We have used cement thus made, and found that it remained on the stock for years. It is not so soft as to run in hot weather, nor so hard as to crack in cold weather.

All of the ingredients for making this cement must be of a good quality.

SOAP-SUDS FOR WATERING PLANTS.

Every one who has a garden, should have all the soap-suds saved to water plants with. It will be found to improve the growth of plants very much.

APPLES.

I have statements without number of the value of

apples for feeding swine. In one case the gain upon raw apples was eleven pounds' weight in twelve days; and in this case nothing except apples was used. The best form of using them seems to be to boil them with potatoes; and it is recommended by several farmers in this case to put the apples at the bottom of the kettle, and the potatoes thus become impregnated with their flavor. This comparatively new use and value of apples may be pronounced a great discovery of the most beneficial character. Many farmers, not accustomed to speak lightly, pronounce them of equal value with potatoes for the fattening of swine, for milk cows, and for beef cattle. I can answer for the human animal. There is no food more healthful or nutritious than apples, cooked or raw. A dish of baked apples and pure milk is of all others most delicious to the unadulterated taste; and the free use of apples and milk in place of the miserable slops of tea and coffee would give to the young bipeds of the family vigorous bodies and bright minds, abate a large item in domestic expenses, and prevent a taste for the two greatest and unalleviated curses with which humanity was ever visited—tobacco and rum.—*Colman's Second Report.*

DIRECTIONS FOR MAKING SWEET CLEAR CIDER THAT SHALL RETAIN ITS FINE VINOUS FLAVOR, AND KEEP GOOD FOR A LONG TIME IN CASKS LIKE WINE.

It is of importance in making cider, that the mill, the press, and all the materials, be sweet and clear, and the straws clear from dust. To make good cider, fruit should be ripe, but not rotten; and when the apples are ground, if the juice is left in the pomace twenty-four hours, the cider will be richer, softer and higher colored. If the fruit is all of the same kind, it is generally thought that the cider will be better, as the fermentation will certainly be more regular, which is of importance. The gathering and grinding of the apples, and the pressing out of the juice, are mere manual labour, performed with very little skill in the operation; but here the great art of making good cider commences; for as soon as the juice is pressed out, nature begins to work a wonderful change in it. The juice of fruit, if left to itself, will undergo three distinct fermentations, all of which change the quality and nature of this fluid. The first is the vinous; the second, the acid, which makes it hard, and prepares it for vinegar: by the third it becomes putrid. The first fermentation is the only one the juice of apples should undergo to make good cider. It is this operation that separates the juice from the filth, and leaves it a clear, sweet, vinous liquor. To preserve it in this state, is the grand secret. This is done by fumigating it with sulphur, which checks any further fermentation, and preserves it in its fine vinous state. It is to be wished that all cider-makers would make a trial of this method. It is attended with no expense, but little trouble, and will have the desired effect. I would recommend that the juice, as it comes from the press, be placed in open-headed casks or vats. In this situation it is most likely to undergo a proper fermentation, and the person attending may with correctness ascertain when this fermentation ceases. This is of great importance, and must be particularly attended to. The fermentation is attended with a hissing noise, bubbles rising to the surface and then forming a soft spongy crust over the liquid. When he crust begins to crack, and white froth appears in the cracks level with the surface of the head, the fermentation is about stopping. At this time the liquor is in a genuine clear state, and must be drawn off immediately into clear casks. This is the time to fumigate it with the sulphur. To do this, take a bit of canvas or rag, about two inches broad and twelve inches long; dip this into melted sulphur, and when a few pails of worked cider are put into the casks, set this match on fire, and hold it in the casks till it is consumed. Then bung the cask and shake it, that the liquor may incorporate with and retain the fumes. After this, fill the cask and bung it up. The cider should be racked off again the latter part of February or first of March; and if not as clear as you wish it, put isinglass into it to fine it, and stir it well. Then put the cask in a cool place, where it will not be disturbed, for the fining to settle. Cider prepared in this manner will keep for years.

It is certainly of great importance to the people of America to cultivate the fruit that is natural to the soil of their country, and to make the most of the fruit which the soil produces, especially when its produce is an article of value and consumption in this country. A Lover of Good Cider.

KERRISON'S RECIPE FOR CIDER.

The following rules for preserving cider, will apply to good cider only, for you cannot preserve bad cider. Let it be made of good sound winter apples, in cool weather, in the month of November or December, and *let no water be mixed with it.* Put it into clean hogsheads, (whiskey hogsheads lately emptied are best), and keep it in a place invariably cool. Fermentation carries off the strength of the cider; therefore prevent it from fermenting as much as possible.

When it exhibits a violent degree of fermentation, put in a half gallon of fourth-proof rectified apple-whiskey; if this does not stop it, put in another half-gallon; the same quantity of pure French brandy will answer better where it can be had. As soon as the fermentation has subsided, and the crude particles settled down, rack it off into a clean hogshead. After this, the cider will undergo a partial fermentation; when it is observed to ferment, and after it has subsided, rack it off again as before. If the crude particles are allowed to remain in the hogshead, they will work up among the cider during every fermentation, and injure it. When it is being racked off, it should be allowed to run with force into a large tub, and pumped from the tub into the hogshead; this serves to break the cider, and is highly beneficial during the first and second racking. Every time it is racked, it must be bunged up tight, and the hogshead kept full; but during the fermentation, the bung should be left out. There are other methods of refining and preserving cider, which are shorter and more certain, but cannot be pursued by farmers with advantage. The above method will be found to answer all domestic purposes.

PERRY.

This is a pleasant liquor, and is made from pears, in the same manner that cider is made from apples. The pears should, in general, be ripe before they are ground. The pulp or pomace should not long remain after grinding, but should immediately be put into the press. The most crabbed and worst eating pears are said to make the best perry. The fruit may be either large or small. The more austere the pears, the better will be the liquor generally. The Taunton Squash pear (cultivated in Massachusetts) produces fruit that is held in the highest estimation in England for perry. It is an early pear, remarkable for the tenderness of its flesh; if it drops ripe from the tree, it bursts from the fall; whence probably its name. The liquor made from it is pale, sweet, remarkably clear, and of strong body, which produces a price in Europe fourfold of common perry. After perry is made, it should be managed in all respects like cider; and must, if necessary, be fined by isinglass. Boiling is said by some to have a good effect on perry, changing it from a white to a flame colored liquor, which grows better by long keeping and bottling. Good perry can scarcely be distinguished from champagne wine; is much lighter, very sparkling, lively, has a pleasanter taste; and is every way worthy of more attention, and of a more extensive manufacture than it at present receives in New England.—*New England Farmer.*

GEOLOGICAL DEFINITIONS.

The primitive earths are four; clay, sand, lime, and magnesia. Clay is called by geologists alumina, alumine, or argillaceous earth. Sand is called silex, silica, siliceous earth, or earth of flints. Lime, as it exists in the soil, is commonly called calcareous earth. The term calcareous is not properly applied to any soil, unless it will effervesce with acids. Each of these earths answers a determinate and specific purpose in the economy and growth of plants, and the perfection of the soil lies in a mixture of the whole. Basis of the whole: the primitive earths which enter into its composition. Vegetable matter: all vegetable substances in a decaying or rotten state.

Animal matter: all animal substances in a putrefying state. Organic matter: a term applied both to animal and vegetable substances in a putrefying state. Vegetable mould: the earthly remains of vegetable substances which have either grown or decayed on the soil, or have been conveyed thither in the progress of cultivation. Loam is a combination of vegetable mould with the primitive earth. Marl is a substance consisting of lime, with a small portion of clay, and sometimes of peat, with a marine 'sand and animal remains. It is useful as a manure, and distinguished by shell, clay, and stone marl.

PROFITS OF COW-KEEPING.

No branch of husbandry is more profitable than the keeping of cows, if properly managed. We have but few farmers in the State of Maine who make great profits by the dairy. Many farmers among us are solicitous to improve their breed of cows, and some raise considerable quantities of good roots, with which to feed during the winter. This is all very good so far; but what is the treatment of cows during the summer season, the time when all, or nearly all, the profits are obtained? Cows kept in short, dry pastures in summer, will not be profitable to their owner, however much ruta baga, mangel-wurzel, or carrots, have been fed out to them during the winter. I believe it to be a fact that cows generally (some few exceptions) are shamefully stinted in their food during summer, in our State, notwithstanding our grazing lands are excellent. I believe that the most profitable mode of keeping cows through the summer is by soiling, or feeding them with grass in the barn or yard. This may frighten some farmers, and excite the ridicule of others; but I think it will be granted, that he is the best farmer who realizes the greatest number of dollars and cents from a given quantity of land with the least amount of labour. Many farmers pride themselves on raising great crops, and one hundred bushels of Indian corn have been raised on a single acre. This is a great profit; but I believe that three thousand bushels of ruta baga may be as cheaply raised, take one year with another, as one hundred bushels of corn. Three thousand bushels of ruta baga will give about a bushel and a half a day each to six cows throughout the whole year. It is easy enough to see that cows fed in this way will be in excellent condition, and yield immense quantities of butter and cheese.

The method of soiling, as described by Dr. Dean, was to feed cows with new mown grass. An acre of rich ground, he says, will summer a number of cows; a little hay or grass will indeed be necessary at all times of the year, but I believe roots should be used in great abundance, and be made the chief article for feeding milch cows throughout the year. Cows do not yield great quantities of milk till June; but by supplying them liberally with roots, they may be made to yield as much milk in March, April, and May, as any part of the year. Farmers, whose cows calve early, and who have abundance of roots, may make prodigious quantities of butter and cheese early in the spring. But how shall the farmer contrive to have a constant supply of roots throughout the summer, and until early root crops are ripe enough for use? This is a question of immense importance. Ruta baga will keep well till July, and is it not possible that by some kind of management this root may be preserved in good condition nearly or quite through the summer? We have an account of an Englishman who buried some potatoes deep in the earth,—so deep that their vegetation was prevented,—and the potatoes, when kept two or three years, were as good flavor and quality as when first ripe. It is believed that potatoes may be kept through the summer without sprouting, in a common ice cellar. It has been contended that potatoes will not sprout where ice will not melt. Chemists pretend to describe the means which nature employs in the process of vegetation, or sprouting. Cannot chemistry tell us how some of those means can be withheld, or so managed, as to prevent, or at least retard the sprouting of vegetables? Would not a summer cellar made air tight answer our purpose? Air is necessary in the process of vegetation, and if we exclude air from vegetables will they sprout? Cannot Yankee ingenuity devise some scheme to prevent vegetables from sprouting during summer? It is to be hoped that some of our enterprising farmers will try various experiments on this subject, as the accomplishment of the object above named would be of immense advantage to every farmer who cultivates roots. If it should be impracticable to preserve roots in good condition throughout the whole summer, I believe that if our farmers practise soiling, they will realize an ample profit by their cows: at the worst, the farmer may have a constant supply of roots for his cows, except about six weeks, from the first of July till the latter part of August; and during this short period he may supply his cows with other food. A steam boiler is of immense advantage to every farmer who cultivates roots. Dr. Dean says that a steam boiler is made by setting a kettle, holding twelve gallons or more, in a furnace made of brick or stone, and over this a hogshead, with one head taken out, and the other bored full of holes. With such a steam boiler a farmer may cook the food for his milch cows with very little fuel, and with very little labor.

Farmers in Europe and in this country have practised soiling their cattle during summer, and those who have had great experience in this mode of summering have declared it to be a much cheaper and more profitable mode than grazing. Much has been said and written of late years in regard to the great profits of root culture; but the farmer who keeps a poor breed of cattle, sheep, and swine, and whose cows in summer range in a short, dry pasture, will never realize great wealth, however great his advantages may be in other respects. The practice of soiling cows in our State would certainly make a great saving of land, and of course it would give to farmers a larger pasture for sheep. More land could be spared for the cultivation of mulberry trees. Immense quantities of manure could be made, especially by those farmers who are not afraid of a little labor in hauling muck, loam, and other materials calculated to absorb the urine of animals, which is most commonly entirely lost.

A STEAM BOILER WORTH HAVING.

T. Fanning, Esq., editor of the Nashville Agriculturist, gives the following account of a steam boiler of his invention.

"I have been studying some time how to construct a cheap and convenient steam boiler, sufficient to cook food for the horses, cattle and swine on my little farm, and I have at length succeeded exactly to my notion.

I purchased a kettle holding sixty gallons, for which I paid $9, and with the labor of two hands for one day I constructed a furnace out of rough lime stone, the cost of which was one dollar more; I then made a box of rough plank three feet square at the bottom, and high enough to hold about ten bushels; the box was perforated with many holes, by the use of a five quarter auger. The bottom of the box is made with plank six feet long, to afford projections to lift it on and off of the kettle. When the cooking process is going on, the top of the box is covered with a piece of carpet, or a close-fitting plank cover to keep in the steam. In using this apparatus, a bushel or two of corn or roots may be put in the kettle, and the box filled with cut oats, corn stocks, turnip tops, beets, potatoes, or anything else that grows on the farm, and the whole may be thoroughly cooked in the course of an hour or two. The machine will not cost more on a farm than the best hand that labors in the field."

CORN STALK SUGAR—DIRECTIONS FOR CULTIVATING THE CORN STALKS, AND MAKING SUGAR.

In various portions of the country, the cultivation of corn for the manufacture of sugar, continues to excite attention. The public are seeking information upon the subject, as the discovery that sugar can be made from the stalk of corn is of recent date. We take pleasure in presenting our readers any facts that may be of importance upon the subject. Dr. Naudin, of Delaware, who has had opportunities to gather knowledge upon the various experiments that have been made, presents some views which will not fail to be regarded with interest.

With regard to the culture, it is stated that 'corn should be planted as broom-corn is commonly planted, very close in the row, probably a stalk every three or four inches. The tillage will be the same as for broom-corn. When the young ears begin to appear, pluck them off carefully, and repeat the gathering as often as necessary, so as to prevent the formation of any grain; because, if grain be allowed to form, it takes all the sugar from the stalk. About the time the corn begins to harden, the making of sugar should begin. It is not necessary to say anything about a proper mill to crush the stalk and separate the juice, because mills of the cheapest kinds only should be employed now, until the business would fully warrant an expensive outlay. It would probably be found that the common cider mill, with plain cylindrical nuts, would be quite sufficient for the farmer who would raise a fourth or half an acre of sugar for his family, and this quantity would be sufficient for a satisfactory experiment.

When the juice is separated from the stalk, about a tablespoonful of whitewash, made of the best quick lime, and about the consistence of thick cream, should be added to each gallon of the juice, and then the boiling should commence. The scum that rises should be carefully removed; and the juice, if this process has been properly conducted, will be quite clear—nearly colorless. Then commences the process of evaporation; and when the juice has boiled down in about the proportion of eight gallons to one, the boiling will be completed, and it may be poured into a shallow tight wooden box to grain.

It has been ascertained, although as yet the reason is not known, that if the juice be boiled in a deep vessel, like the common cooking vessel, sugar will seldom be obtained; while if it be done in a shallow vessel, so that the juice at the commencement of the boiling shall not be more than three to five inches deep, sugar will be obtained without difficulty. It has been ascertained, also, that the sugar from corn will not grain so readily as that from sugar cane. And in some instances, it has remained more than a week after the boiling, before the sugar was formed, and yet excellent sugar was made.

It should be particularly remembered, that the juice should be boiled as soon as separated from the stalk. It becomes acid very soon, and no sugar can be made if the juice be allowed to stand two or three hours before it is boiled. The juice will even spoil in the stalk before it is ground, if the stalk be cut off a few hours before grinding. It is necessary, then, that every part of the process should be done with the greatest despatch. The stalks should be brought to the mill as soon as cut, and ground immediately. The vessel for boiling ought to be properly filled in an hour, or at most two hours, after grinding. And the process of boiling down should immediately commence, and be continued until completed.

Excellent syrup, superior to the best molasses, will be obtained by observing the above directions, and boiling five gallons of juice to one gallon.

The juice of the corn stalk is very rich in sugar, when cultivated in the manner suggested. Tested by Beaume's saccharometer, the instrument used to measure the strength of syrups, the juice of corn stalks weighs 10 to 10 1-2 degrees, which is about the weight of the best cane in the West Indies, and is richer than the juice of the cane in Louisiana, which is seldom heavier than 8 1-2 degrees. One gallon of juice will produce nearly 1 1-4 pounds of sugar; and an acre of good corn will yield, if carefully expressed, from 700 to 1000 gallons of juice.

JAUFFRET'S MODE OF MANUFACTURING MANURE.

We promised, a week or two ago, to give Jauffret's mode of manufacturing manure from straw, weeds, and other vegetable matters. Jauffret is a Frenchman, and has taken out a patent for his mode in France and England, but that cannot hinder the practising his mode in this country, provided he has not also obtained a patent from the United States. The following is a condensed statement of his mode.

The first thing to be done, is to prepare a quantity of what he calls saturated water, which is done by having a vat made of any convenient size, which is half filled with water, and into which is thrown weeds, and almost any kind of vegetable matter that will ferment readily, so as to fill it, with the water, three-fourths full. He then adds, to a vat 12 feet long, six feet wide and six feet deep, ten pounds of quick lime, and five ounces of sal ammoniac. Then you may add sink water, refuse from the kitchen, dead animals, and such like matters. Stir it up occasionally, and if it becomes too offensive in odor, add more unslacked lime occasionally. The next step is to have another vat, smaller than the other, into which sufficient of the above made liquor is to be put to dissolve, or mix with the following materials, which last prepared water he calls Lessive.

Take 200 lbs. of fecal matter and urine (from vaults or privies), 50 lbs. of chimney soot, 400 lbs. of gypsum (plaster of Paris), 60 lbs. of unslacked lime,

20 lbs. of unleached wood ashes, 1 lb. of sea salt, 10 ozs. of saltpetre, 50 lbs. of what he calls leaven of manure. Mix all these with the saturating water till it makes a thick porridge. The leaven of manure is the drainings of a former operation, if there has been one. The above ingredients should be mixed as follows. Stir the first vat up till it is thick, and then pour a portion of it into the lessive vat; into this throw the lime, then the soot, then the ashes, then the fecal matter, the saltpetre. The plaster of Paris is to be thrown in little by little, stirring the mixture to prevent caking. When the whole is well mixed, stir in the leaven.

When the above substances cannot be obtained but at too great expense, Jauffret substitutes other things; for instance:—Instead of fecal matter and urine, take 280 lbs. of horse, cow, or pig dung: for the gypsum, 100 lbs. of baked or burnt earth or clayey loam; for the soot, 100 lbs. sheep manure, and the same weight in mud; for the unleached ashes, 50 lbs. of leached ashes or 2 lbs. of potash; for sea salt, 100 lbs. of sea water. If you come short of lessive, make it up with the saturating water, always using the most impure and putrid that you can obtain.

Having got the above materials ready, clear away a spot of ground and beat it hard, so that water will not soak in readily, and make little pits around this plat into which the liquor which drains from the heap may run. Then take your straw, weeds, &c., or whatever you wish to convert into manure, and put them into a vat of lessive; wet and pack them into a heap, treading them down so as to make them compact. At every layer, of a foot, pour on a quantity of the lessive, and tread it in so that the whole shall be well mixed together. The heap may be six or seven feet high, and when all is packed, spread the bottom of the lessive vat on the top so as to slime it all over, beating and pressing all about so as to make it as snug and compact as possible. At the end of 48 hours a fermentation commences. On the third day the top of the heap is to be opened six inches, and the sediment which was thrown on to the top is turned over, and another drenching is given with the lessive, and again covered up as before. On the seventh day make holes near each other with a fork, say three feet deep, and another drenching given and again covered up. About the ninth day give it another drenching through holes somewhat deeper. In 12 or 15 days the manure will be fit to spread.

It will at once be perceived that it will not do to work upon this in freezing weather. Our readers will also perceive that the principle of manufacturing manure in this way, depends on mixing matters in a putrefying and liquid state, to those which are dry and inert, so as to bring about fermentation among the whole and reduce them to a soluble state; or, as we before expressed it, using a rotten liquor to assist in the decomposition of vegetable matters.

Maine Farmer.

ON PREPARING SEED CORN.

Dissolve saltpetre in water, so as to make it very strong. Soak your seed corn therein, until it becomes swelled; then plant it in the usual way, taking care not to let it be long out of the brine before it is covered. It will produce three times the crop, and will be ripe sooner than the same sort of corn, planted without soaking, on ground of the same quality.

COOKERY

MADE PLAIN AND EASY

WITH A

VALUABLE COLLECTION OF RECIPES IN THE HOUSEHOLD
DEPARTMENT FOR FAMILIES, AND A VALUABLE
COLLECTION OF DOMESTIC RECIPES ON VARIOUS
SUBJECTS AND MATTERS, VERY USEFUL,

WITH AN INDEX.

COLLECTED FROM SOME OF THE BEST LATE AUTHORS, AND
SEVERAL OF THE BEST AGRICULTURAL WORKS.

DOMESTIC RECIPES.

COOKERY.

RECIPE FOR MAKING GOOD BREAD.

James Roche, long celebrated in Baltimore, as a baker of excellent bread, having retired from business, has furnished the Baltimore American with the following recipe for making good bread, with a request that it should be published for the information of the public:

"Take an earthen vessel, larger at the top than the bottom, and in it put one pint of milk-warm water, one and a half pounds of flour, and half a pint of malt yeast; mix them well together, and set it away (in winter it should be in a warm place), until it rises and falls again, which will be in from three to five hours (it may be set at night if wanted in the morning): then put two large spoonsful of salt into two quarts of water, and mix it well with the above rising; then put in about nine pounds of flour and work your dough well, and set it by until it becomes light? Then make it out into loaves. New flour requires one-fourth more salt than old and dry flour. The water also should be tempered according to the weather; in spring and fall it should only be milk-warm; in hot weather, cold; and in winter, warm."

The oven should be made hotter than necessary, and allowed to cool down after being cleared, so that a handful of flour thrown in will not burn, but turn a brown color. The loaves may be formed while trying the temperature of the oven, and be put in soon after. If the loaves are large it will require a little more than an hour to bake them sufficiently.

TO MAKE EXCELLENT BREAD WITHOUT YEAST.

Scald about a double handful of Indian meal, into which put a little salt and as much cold water as will make it rather warmer than new milk. Then stir in wheat flour till it is as thick as a family pudding, and set it down by the fire to rise. In about half an hour it generally draws thin. You may then sprinkle a little fresh flour on the top, and mind to turn the pot around, that it may not bake to the side of it. In three or four hours, if you mind the above directions, it will rise and ferment as if you had set it with top yeast. When it does, make it up in a soft dough, flour a pan, put in your bread, set it before the fire covered up, turn it around to make it equally warm, and in about half an hour it will be light enough to bake.

A SHORT WAY TO MAKE OLD BREAD NEW.

Bread that is several days old may be renewed so as to have all the freshness and lightness of new bread by simply putting it into a common steamer over a fire, and steaming half or three quarters of an hour. The vessel under the steamer containing the water should not be more than half full, otherwise the water may boil up into the steamer, and wet the bread. After the bread is thus steamed, it should be taken out of the steamer, and wrapped loosely in a cloth to dry and cool, and remain so two or three hours, when it will be ready to be cut and used. It will then be like cold new bread. By this process we may work such a change in old bread as will make it in all respects new, except in its deleterious qualities, and thus, at the same time, gratify the taste and subserve the purposes of health and economy. New bread, it is well known, cannot be eaten with perfect impunity until it has undergone the process of ripening; and, indeed, physicians say it ought not, as a general rule, to be eaten till the day after it is made. A way is pointed out above by which a taste for new bread may be gratified without exposure to injury.

SODA BREAD.

A correspondent of the Newry Telegraph gives the following recipe for making soda bread, stating that there is no bread to be had equal to it for invigorating the body, promoting digestion, strengthening the stomach, and improving the state of the bowels. He says: "Put a pound and a half of good wheaten meal (ground with the bran remaining) into a large bowl; mix with it two teaspoonsful of finely powdered salt; then a large spoonful of supercarbonate of soda; dissolve it in half a teaspoonful of cold water, and add to it the meal. Rub up all immediately together. Then pour into the bowl as much sour buttermilk as will make the whole into a soft dough. Then make it into a thin cake or loaf, and put it into a Dutch oven, baking it with a moderate heat till done. Take off the oven lid occasionally to see that it does not burn." This, he concludes, when somewhat cool and moderately buttered, is as wholesome food as ever entered a man's stomach.

DYSPEPSIA BREAD.

The wheat should be of good quality, cleansed from dirt and all impurity, and ground with sharp stones to cut the bran fine. The flour thus prepared, the bread is to be made with good yeast, and baked so as to be light and sweet, which any well skilled housewife knows how to do. Home-made yeast is preferable to brewer's, because the latter often contains poison. The bread should not be eaten under twelve hours after it is baked, for everybody knows that warm bread, cakes, or anything of the kind, is highly injurious.

Bread made as follows, is light and wholesome, and has the sweet and peculiar taste of the wheat in its natural state. Take of the unbolted meal any desirable quantity, and make it into a stiff dough with milk somewhat sour or changed, which has been previously sweetened by the addition of saleratus. It is better to dissolve the saleratus in warm water before it is used, and no more should be put into the milk than is necessary to give it a sweet taste. If any sourness remains in the milk it will cause the bread to be heavy. As soon as the dough is put in the pan, preparatory to baking, plunge a case knife through it to the bottom, cutting across two-thirds of the mass. This prevents the loaf from becoming solid in the middle. The bread will be more light by allowing the dough to stand fifteen or twenty minutes before putting it into the oven.

Bread thus prepared is fit for the table of an emperor, and besides being nourishing and easy of digestion, is one of the best medicines in the world. Persons with the dyspepsia should eat it at every meal.

It excites the secretion of saliva, and leaves the mouth moist, whereas the fine wheat bread often dries the mouth, and can scarcely be swallowed without frequent draughts of tea, coffee, or other drink. It is delicious to the taste, and with new milk boiled, and thickened with fine flour, adding cream if desirable, it makes superior toast, which is excellent for persons recovering from sickness. The bread cut into thin slices and toasted until it is quite hard and brown, makes superior coffee, especially when boiled with sugar and milk. There is no beverage more delicious and nourishing. I know of many families who use it instead of the ordinary tea and coffee, and they find it much better for their health.

TO MAKE POTATOE BREAD.

Boil the potatoes not quite so soft as common, then dry them a short time on the fire, peel them while hot, and mash them as fine as possible; next put a small quantity of pearlash to new yeast; while it is working briskly add as much flour as can be worked in, mix the whole well together, but do not add any water to it. After the dough is thus prepared, let it stand an hour and a half, or two hours, before it is put into the oven: observe, it will not require so long baking as regular flour bread.

RICE FAMILY BREAD.

One quart of rice flour made into a stiff pap by wetting it with warm water, not so hot as to make it lump; when well wet, add boiling water as much as two or three quarts; stir it continually until it boils, then add one pint of milk; when cool enough to avoid scalding, add half a pint of good yeast, and as much wheat flour as will make it of the proper consistency of bread; put it to rise: when sufficiently risen, it will be necessary to add a little more wheat flour. If baked too soft the loaves will be hollow.

TURNIP BREAD.

Let the turnips first be peeled, and boiled in water till soft and tender; then strongly pressing out the juice, mix them together, and when dry (beaten, or pounded very fine), with their weight of wheat meal; mix together, and season as you do other bread, and knead it up thin, letting the dough remain a little to ferment; make the dough into loaves, and bake it like common bread. Some roast turnips in a paper under embers, and eat them with sugar and butter.

PUMPKIN BREAD.

The pumpkin is first deprived of the rind, and afterward cut up into slices and boiled; when soft enough it is strained in a colander and mashed up very fine. In this state it may be used in pies, or mixed with flour for pudding, cake, &c. If it be intended for bread, it may be made up with wheaten flour in the proportion of one-third to half. The sponge must be first set in the ordinary way with yeast in the flour, and the pumpkin worked in as it begins to rise: use as much pumpkin as will bring the dough to a proper degree of stiffness without water. Care should be taken that the pumpkin is not so hot as to scald the leaven. It requires more baking than bread made entirely of wheat.

CORN BREAD.

Stir up one quart of Indian meal with milk, add

two beaten eggs and a tablespoonful of melted butter, pour the batter into a bakepan, and slowly bake either with coals on the lid and setting on them, or hung over the fire. This is a nice process, and upon the baking greatly depends the flavor of the bread. Eaten warm with butter, we have found it the most delicious kind of bread we ever tasted.

LIGHT CORN BREAD.

Stir four pints of meal into three pints of warm water, add one large teaspoonful of salt, let it rise five or six hours, then stir it up with the hand, and bake it in a brisk oven.

Another method is to make mush, and before it gets cold, stir in half a pint of meal. Let it rise, and bake as the first.

YEAST FOR BREAD.

The following method of making yeast for bread is both easy and expeditious. Boil one pound of good flour, a quarter of a pound brown sugar, and a little salt, in two gallons of water, for one hour; when milk-warm, bottle it and cork it close; it will be fit for use in twenty-four hours. One pint of this will make eighteen pounds of bread.

ANOTHER.—Boil twelve clean middle-sized potatoes, and at the same time boil in another vessel a handful of hops in a quart of water. Peel and mash the potatoes fine. Pour part of the hop water while hot upon the potatoes, and mix them well. Then add the remainder of the hop water with a spoonful of sugar; beat all well; add a small portion of yeast to bring on the fermentation, and set it in a cool place. All the utensils must be scalded every time they are used, and washed perfectly clean. One cupful of the above potatoe yeast will answer for two quarts of flour. The above yeast is easily kept, and does not become sour.

MILK YEAST.

Half a pint of milk boiled, cooled with half the quantity of water, or as much as to make it milkwarm, a teaspoonful of salt, and sufficient flour to make a tolerably thin batter. Then put it in a mug with a cover, and set it in a pot of warm water near the fire; when it froths up so as to appear light, it is then fit for use.

TO MAKE NAPLES BISCUIT.

One pound and a half of flour, the same quantity of sugar, nine eggs, half a pint of rose water. Beat the eggs well, put the rose water in by degrees, then mix the flour and sugar together; put it in by degrees.

SUGAR BISCUIT.

Three pounds of flour sifted, one pound of butter, a pound and a half of powdered sugar, half a pint of milk, two tablespoonfuls of brandy, a small teaspoonful of pearlash dissolved in water, four tablespoonsful of caraway seeds; put the butter into the flour, add the sugar and caraway seeds, pour in the brandy, and then the milk, lastly put in the pearlash; stir all well with a knife, and mix it thoroughly till it becomes a lump of dough; flour your paste-board, and lay the dough on it; knead it very well, divide it into eight or ten pieces, and knead each piece separately, then put them all together, and knead them very well in one lump; cut the dough in half and roll it out in sheets about half an inch thick; beat the sheets of dough very hard on both sides with the rolling pin, cut them out into round cakes with the edge of a tumbler, butter the iron pans and lay the cakes in them: bake them of a very pale brown. If done too much, they will lose their taste. These cakes kept in a stone jar, closely covered from the air, will continue perfectly good for several months.

SWEET CRACKERS.

One teacup of coarse wheat meal, one of sour milk or buttermilk, three-fourths of a teacup of sugar, half a teaspoonful of pearlash, well worked, rolled thin, and well baked.

DYSPEPSIA CRACKERS

Can be made with unbolted flour, water and saleratus, that will be much esteemed, and found very convenient for travelling.

GRAHAM WAFERS.

Take one quart of wheat meal, one half pint of Indian meal, and a little salt. Mix them with water, roll them out very thin, and bake them hard. Add a little sugar if you choose.

TO MAKE RICE CRACKERS.

Take a pint of warm water, a teaspoonful of salt, adding a pint of flour, and it will give you two dozen wafers.

TO MAKE RICE CAKES.

Take a pint of soft-boiled rice, a half pint of milk or water, to which add twelve spoonfuls of the rice flour. Divide it into small cakes, and bake them in a brisk oven.

RICE GRIDDLE CAKES.

Boil one large cup of whole rice quite soft in milk, and while hot stir in a little rice flour, or Indian meal. When cold, add two or three eggs and a little salt. Bake in small thin cakes on the griddle.

TO MAKE RICE JOHNNY CAKES.

To three spoonsful of soft boiled rice add a small teacup of water or milk, then add six spoonsful of rice flour, which will make a large johnny cake, or six waffles.

ANOTHER.—Take one quart of milk, three eggs, one teaspoonful of saleratus, one teacupful of wheat flour, and Indian meal sufficient to make a batter of the consistency of pancakes. Bake quick in pan previously buttered, and eat warm with butter or milk. The addition of the wheat flour is found to be a great improvement in the art of making these cakes.

TO MAKE RICE PUFFS.

To a pint of rice flour add a teaspoonful of salt, a pint of boiling water; beat up four eggs, stir them well together; put from two to three spoonsful of fat in a pan, make it boiling hot, and drop a spoonful of the batter into the fat, as you do in making common fritters.

INDIAN MEAL CAKES.

To three pints of Indian meal, add a piece of butter as large as an egg, and a teaspoonful of salt. Put two teacupsful of boiling water, stir it in, then add three eggs, and milk to make it to the consistency of batter. Half a teaspoonful of saleratus.

BUCKWHEAT CAKES.

Put a large spoonful of yeast and a little salt into a quart of buckwheat, in a jar, and make it into a batter with cold water; let it rise well, and bake it on a griddle. It turns sour very quickly, if it be allowed to stand any time after it has risen. They should be buttered, and served up while hot, as they are not good when eaten cold.

ANOTHER.—In the room of water, mix up your butter with buttermilk; instead of leaven or yeast, use a little saleratus (about one teaspoonful to a pint of milk), and two or three eggs. If you do not pronounce them the best buckwheat cakes you ever ate, you and I do not agree in taste.

BATTER CAKES.

One pint of cream, one pint of sour milk or buttermilk, four eggs, a teaspoonful of salt, saleratus sufficient to destroy the acidity of the milk, and three pints of sifted flour, or enough to make a stiff batter. Stir the articles well together, and bake in a deep dish. If for griddle cakes, the batter may be made a little thinner, by not adding so much flour. To be eaten hot with butter.

OYSTER CORN CAKES.

Take one quart of green corn, rasped from the ear with a coarse grater, two teacupsful of new milk, one teacupful of flour, mix them together, and add two eggs well beaten; season the batter with salt and pepper, and bake upon a griddle. The corn should be in a state most suitable for roasting or boiling. The preparation makes a capital dish.

TO MAKE PANCAKES.

Take a quart of milk, beat in six or eight eggs, leaving half the white out; mix it well till your batter is of a proper thickness. You must observe to mix your flour first with a little milk, then add the rest by degrees; put in two spoonfuls of beaten ginger, a glass of brandy, and a little salt; stir all together; make your stew-pan very clean, put in a piece of butter as large as a walnut, then pour in a ladle of batter which will make a pancake, moving the pan round that the batter may be all over the pan: shake the pan, and when you think the under side done enough, turn it, and when both sides are done, lay it in a dish before the fire, and so do with the rest.

WASHINGTON CAKE.

This cake derives its name from the fact that it was a great favorite at the table of General Washington; the last two years of his life, it always formed one of the delicacies of his breakfast-table, and is considered one of the standing dishes of a Virginian.

Take two pounds of flour, one quart of milk, with an ounce of butter, heated together; put the milk and butter into the flour when it is about lukewarm, add one gill good yeast, three eggs, a teaspoonful of salt, place it in pans over night, and bake it in the morning in a quick oven for three-quarters of an hour.

FLANNEL CAKES.

Two pounds of flour, six eggs well beaten, one wineglass of yeast, a little salt, wet with milk into a thick batter, and set it to rise. Bake them in small pans.

TO MAKE CIDER CAKES.

One pound and a half of flour, half a pound of

sugar, a quarter of a pound of butter, half a pint of cider, one teaspoonful of pearlash, spice to your taste. Bake it till it turns easily in the pans—about half an hour.

SPONGE CAKE.

Twelve eggs, ten ounces of sifted flour dried near the fire, a pound of loaf sugar powdered and sifted, twelve drops of essence of lemon, a grated nutmeg, a teaspoonful of powdered cinnamon and mace mixed. Beat the eggs as light as possible. Eggs for sponge or almond cakes require more beating than for any other purpose. Beat the sugar by degrees into the eggs; beat very hard, and continue to beat some time after the sugar is all in. No sort of sugar but loaf will make light sponge cake. Stir in gradually the spice and essence of lemon. Then by degrees put in the flour, a little at a time, stirring around the mixture very slowly with a knife. If the flour is stirred in too hard, the cake will be tough. It must be done lightly and gently, so that the top of the mixture will be covered with bubbles. As soon as the flour is all in begin to bake it, as setting will injure it. Put it in small tins, well buttered, or in one large tin pan. The thinner the pans the better for sponge cake. Fill the small tins about half full. Grate loaf sugar over the top of each before you set them in the oven. Sponge cake requires a very quick oven, particularly at the bottom. It should be baked as fast as possible, or it will be tough and heavy, however light it may have been before it went into the oven. It is of all cakes most liable to be spoiled in baking. When taken out of the tins, the cakes should be spread on a sieve to cool. If baked in one large cake, it should be iced. A large cake of twelve eggs should be baked at least an hour in a quick oven. For small cakes ten minutes are generally sufficient. If they get very much out of shape in baking, it is a sign that the oven is too slow.

POUND CAKE.

Take a pound of butter, beat it in an earthen pan with your hand one way till it is like a fine thick cream; then have ready twelve eggs, put half the whites, beat them well, and beat them up with the butter, a pound of flour beat in it, a pound of sugar, a pound of currants, clean washed and picked, and a few caraways. Beat it all well together for an hour with your hands, or a large wooden spoon: butter a pan and put it in, and then bake it an hour in a quick oven.

TO MAKE GINGERBREAD CAKE.

Take three pounds of flour, one pound of sugar, one pound of butter rubbed in very fine, two ounces of ground ginger, a large nutmeg grated; then take a pound of treacle, a quarter of a pint of cream; make them warm together; by adding a spoonful of saleratus it will improve them: make up the bread stiff, roll it out and make it up into thin cakes, cut them out with a teacup or small glass, or roll them round like nuts, and bake them on tin plates in a slack oven.

SOFT GINGERBREAD, VERY NICE.

Four teacups of flour, two cups of molasses, half a cup of butter, two cups of buttermilk, a cup of thick cream, three eggs, one tablespoonful of ground ginger, and the same of saleratus. Mix them all together, with the exception of the buttermilk, in which the saleratus must be dissolved, and then added to the rest. It must not stand long before sent to bake.

COMMON GINGERBREAD.

A quart of molasses, one pound of fresh butter, two pounds and a half of flour sifted, a pint of milk, a small teaspoonful of pearlash, or saleratus, a teacupful of ginger; cut the butter into the flour, add the ginger; having dissolved the pearlash in the milk, stir the milk and molasses alternately into the other ingredients; stir it very hard for a long time, till it is quite light: put some flour on your paste-board, take out small portions of the dough, and make it with your hand into long rolls; then curl up the rolls into round cakes; or twist two rolls together, or lay them in straight lengths or sticks side by side, and touching each other: put them carefully in buttered pans, and bake them in a moderate oven, not hot enough to burn them. You can, if you choose, cut out the dough with tins, in the shape of hearts, circles, ovals, &c., or you may bake it all in one, and cut it into squares when cold. If the mixture appears too thin, add gradually a little more sifted flour.

JUMBLES.

Three eggs, half a pound of flour sifted, half a pound of butter, half a pound of powdered loaf sugar, a tablespoonful of rosewater, a nutmeg grated, a teaspoonful of mace and cinnamon; stir the butter and sugar to a cream, beat the eggs very light, and throw them all at once into the pan of flour; then put in the butter and sugar, and add the spice and rosewater. If you have no rosewater, six or seven drops of strong essence of lemon will answer, or more if the essence be weak: stir the whole very hard, and flour your hands well: take up with your knife a portion of the dough, and lay it on the board; roll it lightly with your hands into long thin rolls, which must be cut into equal lengths, curled up into rings, and laid gently into an iron or tin pan, buttered, not too close to each other, as they spread in baking. Bake them in a quick oven about five minutes, and grate loaf sugar over them when cool.

MRS. G.'S FAMOUS BUNNS.

One pound and a half of flour (a quarter of a pound left to sift in last), half a pound of butter cut up fine together; then add four eggs; beat up to a high froth four teacups of milk, half a wine glass of brandy, wine, and rose water, each, and one wine glass of yeast. Stir it all together with a knife, and add half a pound of sugar. Then sift in the quarter of a pound of flour, and when the lumps are all beaten fine, set them to rise in the pans they are to be baked in. This quantity will make four square pans full.

RUSK.

A quarter of a pound of powdered sugar, a quarter of a pound of fresh butter, one pound of flour sifted, one egg, three wine glasses of milk, a wine glass and a half of the best yeast, a tablespoonful of rosewater, a teaspoonful of powdered cinnamon. Sift your flour into a pan, cut up the butter in the milk, and warm them a little, so as to soften the butter, and not to melt it entirely. Beat your egg; pour the milk and butter into your pan of flour, then the egg, then the rosewater and spice, and, lastly, the yeast. Stir all well together with a knife. Spread some flour on your paste-board, lay the dough on it, and knead it well.

Then divide it into small pieces of an equal size, and knead each piece into a little thick round cake. Butter your iron pan, lay the cakes in it, and set them in a warm place to rise. Prick the tops with a fork. When they are quite light bake them in a moderate oven.

CORN MEAL RUSK.

Take six cupsful of corn meal, four of wheat flour, two cupsful of molasses, and one teaspoonful of saleratus; mix the whole together, and knead into dough; then make two cakes. Bake them as you would pone for three-fourths of an hour, and you will have one of the most grateful descriptions of bread that ever graced the table.

ROLLS.

Three pints of flour sifted, two teaspoonsful of salt, four tablespoonsful of the best brewer's yeast, or six of home-made-yeast, a pint of luke-warm water, half a pint more of warm water, and a little more flour to mix in before the kneading. Mix the salt with the flour, and make a deep hole in the middle. Stir the warm water into the yeast, and pour it into the hole in the flour. Stir it with a spoon just enough to make a thin batter, and sprinkle some flour over the top. Cover the pan, and set it in a warm place for several hours. When it is light add half a pint more of luke-warm water, and make it, with a little more flour, into a dough. Knead it very well for ten minutes. Then divide it into small pieces, and knead it separately. Make it into round cakes or rolls. Cover them, and set them to rise about an hour and a half. Bake them, and when done let them remain in the oven, without the lid, for about ten minutes.

SOFT MUFFINS.

Five eggs, a quart of milk, two ounces of butter, a teaspoonful of salt, two large tablespoonsful of brewer's yeast, or four of home-made yeast, and enough of sifted flour to make a stiff batter. Warm the milk and butter together, add to them the salt. Beat the eggs very light, and stir them into the milk and butter. Then stir in the yeast, and lastly sufficient flour to make a thick batter. Cover the mixture, and set it to rise in a warm place about three hours. When it is quite light, grease your baking iron and your muffin rings. Set the rings on the iron, and pour the batter into them. Bake them a light brown. When you split them to butter, do not cut them with a knife, but pull them open with your hands. Cutting them while hot will make them heavy.

DOUGHNUTS.

To one pound of flour put one quarter of a pound of butter, one quarter of a pound of sugar, and two spoonsful of yeast; mix them all together in warm milk or water, to the thickness of bread; let it rise, and make them in what form you please; boil your lard, and put them in.

CRULLERS.

Ten eggs, one pound and a half of sugar, three-fourths of a pound of butter, one teacup of milk, one teaspoonful of saleratus, spice to your taste, and flour enough to make soft dough—let your lard be boiling, then make them into what shape you please and put them in.

THE FLOATING ISLAND—A PRETTY DISH FOR THE MIDDLE OF A TABLE AT A SECOND COURSE, OR FOR SUPPER.

You may take a soup dish, according to the size and

quantity you would make, but a pretty deep glass is best, and set into a china dish: first take a quart of the thickest cream you can get, make it pretty sweet with fine sugar, pour on a gill of sack, grate in it the yellow rind of a lemon, and mill the cream until it is all of a thick frost; then carefully pour the thin from the froth into a dish; take a French roll, or as many as you want; cut it as thin as you can; lay a layer of that as light as possible on the cream; then a layer of currant jelly, then a very thin layer of roll, and then hartshorn jelly, then French roll, and over that whip your froth which you saved of the cream, very well milled up, and lay it at top as high as you can heap it; and as for the rim of the dish, set it round with fruit and sweetmeats according to your fancy. This looks very pretty in the middle of the table, with candles round, and you may make it of as many different colors as you can fancy, and according to what jellies and jams or sweetmeats you have; or at the bottom of your dish you may put the thickest cream you can get, but that is as you fancy.

KISSES.

One pound of the best loaf sugar, powdered and sifted. The whites of four eggs. Twelve drops of essence of lemon. A teacup of currant jelly. Beat the whites of four eggs till they stand alone. Then beat in, gradually, the sugar, a teaspoonful at a time. Add the essence of lemon, and beat the whole very hard.

Lay a wet sheet of paper on the bottom of a square tin pan. Drop on it, at equal distances, a little of the beaten egg and sugar, and then add on each, a small teaspoonful of stiff currant jelly. Then with a large spoon, pile some of the beaten egg and sugar on each lump of jelly, so as to cover it entirely. Drop on the mixture as evenly as possible, so as to make the kisses of a round smooth shape.

Set them in a cool oven, and as soon as they are colored, they are done. Then take them out and place them two bottoms together. Lay them lightly on a sieve, and dry them in a cool oven, till the two bottoms stick fast together, so as to form one ball or oval.

RICE MILK FOR A DESSERT.

Boil half a pint of rice in water till tender. Pour off the water, and add a pint of milk, with two eggs beaten and well stirred into it. Boil all together for a few minutes. Serve it up hot, and eat it with butter, sugar, and nutmeg. It may be sweetened and cooled in moulds, turned out on a deep dish, and surrounded with rich milk, seasoned with wine and sugar.

APPLE CUSTARDS.

To one pound of apples stewed, in a saucepan, add three quarters of a pound of good brown sugar, half a pound of butter, with eight eggs beat up and mixed together, with a little cinnamon or nutmeg grated. Take plates and put on your bottom crust. Fill up, and bake as other pies and tarts.

PLAIN CUSTARDS.

A quart of rich milk, eight eggs, a quarter of a pound of powdered sugar, with a nutmeg grated fine. Beat the eggs very light, and stir them gradually into the milk. Bake it in cups—when cool, grate nutmeg over the top.

TO MAKE A NORFOLK DUMPLING.

Make a thick batter, as you would for pancakes; take half a pint of milk, two eggs, a little salt, and make it into a batter with flour; have ready a clean saucepan of water boiling, into which drop the batter. Be sure the water boils fast, and two or three minutes will boil them; then throw them into a sieve or colander to drain the water away; then turn them into a dish and stir a lump of fresh butter into them; eat them hot, and they are very good.

TO MAKE AN APPLE DUMPLING.

Take a good puff paste, pare some large apples, cut them into quarters and take out the cores very nicely; take a piece of crust and roll it round enough for one apple: if they are large they will not look well, so roll the crust round each apple and make them round like a ball with a little flour in your hand; have a pot of water boiling, take a clean cloth, dip it in the water and shake flour over it; tie each dumpling by itself, and put them in the water boiling all the time, and if your crust is light and good, and the apples not too large, half an hour will boil them, but if the apples are large they will take an hour boiling. When they are boiled enough, take them up and lay them in a dish and send them to the table; have good fresh butter melted with sugar mixed for sauce.

TO MAKE APPLE FRITTERS.

Beat the yolk of eight eggs, and the whites of four well together, and strain them into a pan; then take a quart of cream, make it as hot as you can bear your fingers in it; when it is cool put in your eggs, beating it well together, then put in nutmegs, ginger, salt, and flour to your liking. Your batter should be pretty thick, then put in apples sliced, and fry them in butter quick.

TO MAKE AN APPLE PUDDING.

Take twelve large apples, pare them and take out the cores, put them into a saucepan with four or five spoonsful of water, boil them till they are soft and thick, then beat them well; stir in a pound of loaf sugar, the juice of three lemons, the yolks of eight eggs beat; mix all well together, bake it in a slack oven, when it is near done throw over a little fine sugar: you may bake it with a puff paste in pans, as you do other puddings or pies.

INDIAN PUDDING.

Take one quart of corn meal, two quarts of warm milk, about blood heat, two teaspoonsful of salt, one teacup of molasses ,or four tablespoonsful of sugar, one tablespoonful of chopped suet, and half a grated nutmeg. Bake in a pan two hours.

ANOTHER, equally excellent.—Take fourteen tablespoonsful of Indian meal, two quarts of boiling milk, two teaspoonsful of salt, and half a tablespoonful of chopped suet. A richer pudding is made by substituting for the fourteen tablespoonsful of Indian meal, seven eggs and seven tablespoonsful of meal. Bake in pans as above two hours.

The sauce may consist of one pint of water, four tablespoonsful of sugar, of butter the size of half an egg, one tablespoonful of vinegar, one tablespoonful of flour, and a quarter of a nutmeg. It should be boiled three or four minutes.

PAIN INDIAN PUDDING.—BAKED.

Scald a quart of milk (skimmed milk will do), and

stir in seven tablespoonsful of sifted Indian meal, a teacupful of molasses, and a large spoonful of ginger, or sifted cinnamon. Bake three or four hours. If whey is wanted in the pudding, pour in a little cold milk after it is all mixed.

RICH INDIAN PUDDING.—BAKED.

Boil a quart of milk, add a pint of fine Indian meal. Stir it well. Mix three tablespoonsful of wheat flour with a pint of milk, so as to have it free from lumps. Mix this with the meal, and stir the whole well together. When the whole is moderately warm, stir in three eggs well beat, with three spoonsful of sugar. Add two teaspoonsful of salt, two of ground cinnamon, or grated nutmegs, and two tablespoonsful of melted butter. When the pudding has baked five or six minutes, stir in half a pound of raisins seeded; and add half a pint of milk for them, as they will render it too dry. Bake three or four hours.

INDIAN PUDDING.—BOILED.

Make a stiff batter by stirring Indian meal into a quart of boiling milk or water. Then stir in two tablespoonsful of flour, three of sugar, half a spoonful of ginger, or two teaspoonsful of cinnamon, and two teaspoonsful of salt, two tablespoonsful of fine chopped suet. Such puddings require a long boiling, say seven or eight hours. They require good sauce for eating.

TO MAKE GREEN-CORN PUDDING.

Gather the corn in the milk, when neither too young nor too ripe. Shell, cut, or scrape the corn from the cob, and pound it fine in a mortar. To four dozen ears add one pint of milk and half a pound of sugar—the whole to be mixed together, and baked about two hours, till the crust shows a dark brown color. It is to be eaten with fresh butter, to which same add a sprinkling of pepper.

POTATOE PUDDING.

One pound of butter, one pound of sugar, beat to a cream; one pound of Irish potatoes, boiled and passed through the colander, eight eggs well beaten, one glass of brandy, one of wine, half a glass of rosewater, and one teaspoonful of spice. Put a bottom crust of puff paste, and bake in deep plates, or dishes.

SWEET POTATOE PUDDING.

Boil one pound of sweet potatoes very tender; rub them while hot through a colander; add six eggs well beaten, three quarters of a pound of powdered sugar, three quarters of a pound of butter, and some nutmeg and lemon-peel, with a glass of brandy; put a bottom crust in the dish, and when the pudding is done sprinkle the top.

PUMPKIN PUDDING.

Half a pound of butter, half a pound of sugar, beat to a cream; one pound of pumpkin stewed and passed through the colander; four eggs, well beaten, one wine glass of brandy, wine, and rosewater, and one teaspoonful of spice; put a bottom crust, and bake in deep dishes.

CARROT PUDDING.

Grate half a pound of carrots, one pound of bread, the whites of eight eggs well beaten, half a pound of butter, half a pint of cream or milk, half a pint of wine and rosewater, and spice; sweeten to taste. Lay a puff paste over the dish. Bake one hour, and sift sugar over it.

TO MAKE PAP PUDDING.

To a quart of milk, add a pint of rice flour; boil it to a pap; beat up six eggs, to which add six spoonsful of Havana sugar, and a spoonful of butter, which, when well beaten together, add to the milk and flour. Grease the pan in which it is to be made. Grate nutmeg over the mixture, and bake it. Rice cakes or puddings are the better for eating warm.

TRANSPARENT PUDDING.

Beat eight eggs very light, add half a pound of pounded sugar, the same of fresh butter melted, and half a nutmeg grated. Set it on a stove, and keep stirring till it is as thick as buttered eggs. Put a puff paste in a shallow dish; pour in the ingredients, and bake it half an hour in a moderate oven. Sift sugar over it, and serve it up hot.

TO MAKE A BATH PUDDING.

Take one pint of new milk, six eggs beat well in the milk, four tablespoonsful of fine flour, three tablespoonsful of yeast, three spoonsful of rosewater, and three spoonsful of Malaga wine, grate into it a small nutmeg, sweeten with fine sugar to your taste; mix them all well together, and let them stand one hour before they are to be baked: bake them in eight small patty-pans, and one large one for the middle of the dish: butter the patty-pans, put them in a fierce oven, and in fifteen minutes they will be done.

TO MAKE A QUAKING PUDDING.

Take a pint of good cream, six eggs, and half the

whites, beat them well and mix with the cream, grate in a small nutmeg, add a little rosewater if it be desired, grate in the crust of a small loaf of bread, or add a spoonful or two of flour first mixed with a little of the cream, or a spoonful of the flour of rice, which you please; butter a cloth well and flour it, then put in your mixtures, tie it not too close, and boil it half an hour: be sure the water boils before you put it in.

TO MAKE A BREAD PUDDING.

Take the crumbs of a small loaf of bread, and as much flour, the yolks of four eggs and two whites, a teaspoonful of ginger, half a pound of raisins seeded, half a pound of currants clean washed and picked, and a little salt; mix first the bread and flour, ginger, salt, and sugar to your taste, then the eggs and as much milk as will make it like a good batter; butter the dish, pour it in and bake it.

RICH BREAD AND BUTTER PUDDING.

Cut a pound loaf of good bread into thin slices. Spread them with butter as for eating. Lay them in a pudding dish; sprinkle between each layer of bread seeded raisins, and citron cut fine. Beat eight eggs with four tablespoonsful of rolled sugar, mix them with three pints of milk, and half a grated nutmeg. Turn the whole on the bread in the pan, and let it remain till the bread has taken up full half the milk; then bake about three-quarters of an hour.

PLUM PUDDING.

Beat eight eggs very light; add one pint of milk, one quart of flour, and three-quarters of a pound of butter, after it has creamed; cut and stone half a pound of raisins, mix them in with the batter, with half a nutmeg grated. Wet your cloth; tie it up tight. Put your pudding in when the water is boiling; shake and stir it for a minute or two, to keep the raisins from settling at the bottom. Boil two hours.

A CAROLINA RICE PUDDING.

Take half a pound of rice; wash it clean; put it into a sauce-pan with a quart of milk; keep stirring it till it is very thick; take great care it does not burn; then turn it into a pan, and grate some nutmeg into it; add two teaspoonsful of beaten cinnamon and a little lemon peel made fine. Mix all together with the yolks of three eggs, and sweeten to your taste. Then tie up close in a cloth, put it into boiling water, and be sure to keep it boiling all the time—an hour and a quarter will be sufficient. Melt butter, and pour over it, and throw some fine sugar all over it. A little wine in the sauce will be a great addition to it.

ANOTHER.—Take a quart of milk; add a pint of flour; boil them to a pap; beat up six eggs, to which add six spoonsful of Havana sugar, and a spoonful of butter, which, when well beaten together, add to the milk and flour. Grease the pan it is to be made in. Grate nutmeg over the mixture, and bake it.

RULES TO BE OBSERVED IN MAKING PUDDINGS.

The outside of a boiled pudding often tastes disagreeable, which arises from the cloth not being nicely washed, and kept in a dry place. It should be dipped in boiling water, squeezed dry, and floured when to be used. If a bread pudding, it should be tied loose ; if a batter pudding, tie it close. The water should boil quick when the pudding is put in, and it should be moved about for a minute or two, lest the ingredients should not mix. Batter puddings should be strained through a coarse sieve when all is mixed. Where a pudding is baked, the pans and basins should be always buttered.

Very good puddings may be made without eggs, but they must have as little milk as will mix, and they must boil three or four hours. A spoonful or two of yeast will answer instead of eggs.

TO MAKE MINCE PIES.

Take beef tongue, weighing about three pounds, cut off the root, wash it perfectly clean, and boil it till it becomes tender ; skin it, and when cold, chop it very finely. Or, if preferred, three pounds of the inside of a sirloin of beef, boiled till it becomes tender, and chopped finely as the other. Mince, as small as possible, two pounds of fresh beef suet ; two pounds of currants, nicely picked, washed, rubbed, and dried at the fire ; two dozen large apples, pared and chopped very fine ; one pound of good brown sugar ; sift half an ounce of mace, and a quarter of an ounce of cloves ; grate in two nutmegs. The grated rind and juice of a large lemon may be added, with a little citron. Put all together into a large pan, and mix it well together with half a pint of good French brandy, and if not moist enough, good sweet cider may be added. Put it down close into a jar, covered closely, and it will be good four months. When you make your pies, take small round dishes, or soup-plates ; lay a thin crust all over them, put in your meat, lay over the crust, and bake them nicely. These pies eat finely cold. If the meat is not used immediately, the apples had better not be put in until wanted.

TO MAKE PUMPKIN PIES.

Take one quart of stewed and strained pumpkin; add one quart of new milk, half a pint of cream, and four eggs well beaten. Mix, and add a little ginger, cinnamon, and sugar, to taste. Put a bottom crust of puff paste, and bake in deep dishes.

ANOTHER.—To one quart of stewed and strained pumpkin, add one quart of new milk, and sweeten to taste. For the crust, take wheat flour; wet with buttermilk to a sufficient stiffness to roll out. Bake it in deep dishes.

ANOTHER.—Take a brown earthen pan, grease it, and sift Indian meal over it, about the thickness of a a quarter of an inch. Prepare the pumpkin in good new milk, and sweeten to taste, and add a little ground rice instead of eggs, with a little ginger. Bake as above.

TO MAKE AN APPLE PIE.

Make a good puff-paste crust; lay some around the sides and bottom of the dish; pare and cut your apples, and stew them; put in a thick layer of apples; throw in half the sugar you design for your pie; make a little orange peel fine; squeeze and throw over them a little of the orange juice, then a few cloves, then the rest of your apples and sugar. You must sweeten to your taste. Boil the peelings and cores of the apples in fair water, with a blade of mace, till it is very good. Strain it, and boil the syrup with a little sugar, till there is but very little, and that good. Pour it into your pie, put on your upper crust, and bake it.

CRANBERRY PIES.

Wash and stew a quart of good sound cranberries; strain them through a coarse sieve; add half a pound of good sugar. Put on a bottom crust in your patty-pans, and fill them up, and bake in a moderate oven for half an hour.

RHUBARB PIES.

Cut the stalks to pieces of the size of a gooseberry, stew them a little in a sauce-pan, put them into a dish with its bottom covered with a crust; squeeze over them a little lemon juice, adding orange-peel, sugar, rose-water, and cinnamon to your taste; cover the whole with a good puff-paste, and then bake it.

SWEET POTATOE PIE.

Select four or five of the largest potatoes; wash them clean; slice them thin, and put in a pan with a puff paste crust, first a layer of potatoes; then season with allspice, cinnamon, sugar, and butter, and so fill up the pan, observing to put a little of the seasoning between each layer as you fill up; one good sized lemon may be cut and sliced thin, and added between each layer of the potatoes, with the other seasoning. A sufficient quantity of water must be added, so that the pie may be moist after it is baked. Cover the top with a puff paste, and bake in an oven.

TOMATO PIES.

The tomatoes are skinned and sliced, and after being

mixed with sugar, spice, and cinnamon to taste, are baked with a puff paste as other pies.

OYSTER PIE.

A hundred large fresh oysters, or more if small, the yolk of six eggs boiled hard, a large slice of stale bread grated, a teaspoonful of salt, a tablespoonful of mixed nutmeg, and cinnamon. Take a large round dish, butter it, and spread a puff paste round the sides, but not at the bottom. Drain off part of the liquor from the oysters, put them into a pan, and season them with pepper, salt, and spice; stir them well with the seasoning. Have ready the yolks of the eggs, chopped fine, and the grated bread. Pour the oysters with the liquor into the dish with the puff paste: strew over them the chopped egg and grated bread, roll out the lid of the pie and put it on. Bake the pie in a quick oven.

CHICKEN PIE.

Parboil and cut up neatly two young chickens. Take the water in which they have been boiled to make a gravy, put into it pepper and salt, and a thickening of flour and butter. Mkae a puff paste crust, and cover your pan. Boil six eggs hard, and put the yolks, cut in two, into the pie, along with the chickens; a few oysters might be laid round among the chickens. Fill the pan with the gravy, and cover with a thick crust. It will require about an hour and a half to bake.

TO MAKE A PIGEON PIE.

Make a puff paste crust, cover your dish, let your pigeons be nicely picked and clean, cut them up and lay them in your pan, and season with pepper, and salt, and put in a good piece of fresh butter, add the yolk of two eggs, and a beef steak in the middle; put as much water as will almost fill the dish, and lay on the top crust and bake it well.

TO MAKE A MUTTON PIE.

Take a loin of mutton, pare off the skin and fat of the insides, cut it into steaks, season it with pepper and salt, to your taste, lay it in a dish or pan, with a crust, and fill it; pour in as much water as will almost fill the dish; then put over a crust, and bake it well.

PORK PIE.

Make a common pie crust, put in a pan, take pork and cut it into small pieces, and beat them a little; season with pepper and salt; fill your pie; put on the top crust, and bake it two hours, with paper over it to prevent it from burning. There should be some gravy in it when done. Veal and lamb pie can be made in the same way.

TO MAKE CHOWDER—(A SEA DISH).

Take a belly-piece of pickled pork, slice it small, and lay them at the bottom of the kettle, strew over it onions, and other sweet herbs agreeable to fancy. Take a middling large cod, slice it small, and season it with pepper, salt, and spice, and flour it a little; make a layer with part of the slices, upon that a slight layer of pork again, and on that a layer of biscuit, and so on, pursuing the like rule until the kettle is filled to about four inches; cover it with nice paste, pour-in about a pint of water, cover the kettle, and keep it over a slow fire about four hours.

TO MAKE PURLOW.

It is a dish made with whole rice, thus:—Instead of plain water boil a piece of bacon, or sound salted pork, and one or two fowls, in the usual way. Take them out, and set them by the fire. Then reduce the water in the pot to the proper quantity for boiling. Add a little salt, spice, and black pepper to the taste, and when boiling put in the rice after well washing. Boil from twenty to thirty minutes. Put the pot then to soak or steam over a few coals, and in twenty minutes the rice will be done. Serve it on a large dish, the bacon or pork and fowls side by side on the top of the rice.

PEARL BARLEY AS A SUBSTITUTE FOR RICE.

It is equally advantageous to the public to learn the use of a known substance, as the discovery of a new one. I am sure the application of barley to another branch of domestic cookery will not be disregarded by some of your readers. I can assure them that they will find it an excellent substitute for rice. It has been long used in this country in soup; and when boiled with milk, sometimes called Scotch rice; but by far the best way of using it is by pounding it in a mortar. In this form it fairly rivals manacroop, tabico, or ground rice, and can be easily procured at one-tenth the price of the first, and one-third of the price of the last substance. It was resorted to as a change of food for my children's breakfast, and the great similarity to manacroop induced us to try it in a pudding for them, and I can assure you, I think it one of the best of the kind. Some management as with either of the other, milk, eggs, &c. What we call pearl barley is the kind used, but I dare say any of the kind would answer.

ANOTHER.—Boil salsify, or vegetable oysters, till the skin will come off easily. When you have taken it off neatly, cut the roots in bits as long as an oyster; put into a deep vegetable dish a layer of crumbs of bread or crackers, a little salt and pepper, and nutmeg, and a covering of butter as thin as you can cut it; then a layer of oysters, till your dish is filled, having crumbs at top. Fill the dish with water, and brown them handsomely. They can remain two hours in the oven without injury, or be eaten in half an hour.

HOW TO BOIL RICE.

Put your rice into an open pot; then cover the rice with water, and put it on the fire to boil. Suffer it to remain on the fire until the rice is soft, which you can ascertain by means of a wooden ladle. Then take it off, and draw off the water, and put a cover on the pot; then place it on coals or hot ashes, and leave it to steam or soak for fifteen or twenty minutes.

COOKING SALSIFY, OR VEGETABLE OYSTER.

1st. Boil the salsify, scrape them, cut them in half lengthwise, dip them in rich batter, and fry them in lard.

2d. Boil the salsify, wash them in a piggin, as potatoes are washed; then put in batter, adding a large teaspoonful of ground ginger, mix it well, and fry it in little patties.

3d. Boil the salsify, and then slice them crosswise, put them in a sauce-pan with a little butter, a spoonful or two of cream, a little pepper, and some salt; stir it till it is of a light brown.

COOKING THE PURPLE EGG PLANT OR GUINEA SQUASH.

Select the squashes, or fruit, when at maturity; cut them into slices, and parboil them in a stewpan; when softened, drain off the water; they may then be fried in batter, made with wheaten flour and an egg, or in fresh batter, with bread grated fine, seasoned before it is put in the pan, with pepper, salt, thyme, and such other herbs as may best suit the taste. Some use marjoram, summer savory, parsley, and onions.

OKRA SOUP.

The pods are of a proper size when two or three inches long, but may be used as long as they remain tender, which is judged of by their brittleness; if good (that is, fit for use), they will snap asunder at the ends, but if they merely bend they are too old, have become woody, and must be rejected; for a few of such pods will spoil a dish of soup. I have taken definite quantities, so that the proper portions of each may be clearly understood by you: smaller quantities may be used, but the proportions ought to be observed, as well as the length of time for boiling.

Take one peck of okra pods, which must be very tender, and of which you will judge by the rule already given; cut them across into very thin slices, not exceeding one-eighth of an inch in thickness, but as much thinner as possible, as the operation is accelerated by their thinness; to this quantity of okra add about one-third of a peck of tomatoes, which are first peeled and cut into pieces. This quantity can be either increased or diminished, as may suit the taste of those for whom it is intended. A coarse piece of beef (a shin is generally made use of) is placed in a digester, with about two and a half gallons of water, and a very small quantity of salt. It is permitted to boil for a few minutes, when the scum is taken off, and the okra and tomatoes thrown in.

These are all the ingredients absolutely necessary, and the soup thus made is remarkably fine. We, however, usually add some corn cut off from the tender roasting ears: the grains from three ears will be enough for the above quantity: we sometimes take about half a pint of Lima beans. Both of these improve the soup, but not so much as to make them indispensable; so far from it, that few add them. The most material thing to be attended to is the boiling, and the excellence of the soup depends almost entirely on this being faithfully done: for, if it be not boiled enough, however well the ingredients may have been selected, the soup will be very inferior, and give little idea of the delightful flavour it possesses when properly done. I have already directed that the ingredients be placed in a digester. This is decidedly the best vessel for boiling this or any other soup, but should there be no digester, then an earthen pot should be prepared; but on no account make use of an iron one, as it would turn the whole soup perblack; the proper colour being green, coloured with the rich yellow of the tomatoes.

The time which is usually occupied in boiling okra soup is five hours. We put it on at 9 A.M., and take it off about 2 P.M., during the whole of which time it is kept boiling briskly; the cook at the same time stirring it frequently and mashing the different ingredients. By the time it is taken off it will be reduced to about one half; but as on the operation of the boiling being well and faithfully executed depends its goodness (as I have already remarked), I will state the criterion by which this is judged of:—the meat separates entirely from the bone, being done to rags; the whole appears as one homogeneous mass, in which none of the ingredients are seen distinct; the object of this long boiling being thus to incorporate them, its consistence should be about that of thick porridge.

TO MAKE CALF'S HEAD SOUP.

Take a calf's head, part of the liver and lights, boil it in six quarts of water, until you can take the bones out, put it on a dish, season it with pepper, salt, and sweet marjoram, thyme and sage, mace and cloves; skim the water, if there be any fat on it; then put it all back in the same water that it was boiled in, and let it boil till done. Just before you take it up put a glass of wine in it, with a little burnt sugar; thicken it with a little butter and flower.

If you wish to make a great deal of soup, you must add a knuckle of veal, as the head only will not make it rich enough. If you wish to make the dish without soup, boil the head in the same way, and season it in the same manner in the dish, with a little of the water it was boiled in; thicken it a little with butter and flour: put it in the oven till you think it is done.

HOW TO COOK GREEN PEAS.

The common method of cooking this delicious vegetable, by boiling in water, is nearly destructive to its flavour, at least so says a lady who has sent us the following method of preparing them for the table, which, after experience, we must add, is a great improvement: " Place in the bottom of your sauce-pan, or boiler, several of the outside leaves of lettuce; put your peas in the dish with two ounces of butter in proportion to half a peck of peas; cover the pan or boiler close, and place over the fire; in thirty minutes they are ready for the table. They can either be seasoned in the pan or taken out. Water extracts nearly all the delicious quality of the green pea, and is as fatal to their flavour as it is destructive to a mad dog.

CALF'S FEET JELLY.

Boil your feet in water sufficient to make them tender, and until they are broken, and the water half wasted; strain it, and when cold take off the fat, and remove the jelly from the sediment, then put it into a sauce-pan with sugar, raisins, wine, lemon-juice, to your taste, and some lemon-peel: when the flavour is rich, put to it the whites of five eggs well beaten; set the sauce-pan on the fire, but do not stir the jelly after it begins to warm. Let it boil twenty minutes after it rises to a head, then pour it through a flannel jelly bag, first dipping the bag in hot water to prevent waste, and squeezing it quite dry: run the jelly through and through until quite clean, then put it into glass jars, or tumblers.

The following mode will greatly facilitate the clearing of jelly:—When the mixture has boiled twenty minutes, throw in a teacupful of cold water; let it boil five minutes longer, then take the sauce-pan off the fire, covered close, and keep it half an hour; after which it will be so clear as to need only once running through the bag, and much waste will be saved. Observe, feet for all jellies are boiled so long by the people who sell them, that they are less nutritious; they should only be scalded to take off the hair. The liquor will require greater care in removing the fat, but the jelly will be far stronger, and of course allow more water.

TO MAKE SAUSAGES.

Take three pounds of nice pork fat and lean together, chop it as fine as possible, season it with a teaspoonful of beaten pepper, and two of salt, some sage made fine, about three spoonsful; mix it well together, have the guts very nicely cleaned, and fill them or put the meat down in a pot. Beef will make good sausages.

ANOTHER.—Twelve pounds of meat, seven pounds of fat from the back of the chine, five spoonsful of salt, six spoonsful of sage, two of thyme, three of pepper; when put into guts, put it into large stone jars, and pour warm milk over it, until the jars are full.

OXFORD SAUSAGES.

The following recipe for making the celebrated Oxford sausages, so much desiderated by the lovers of good eating in England, is from a late English publication.

Ingredients: one pound and a half of pig meat without any skin, and a half pound of veal. One pound and a half of beef suet, the yolks and whites of five eggs. A dessert-spoonful of sifted sage, after being well dried. Pepper and salt to the taste.

HOW TO MAKE THE ABOVE INTO SAUSAGES.

Chop the meat small, and then pound it together in a marble mortar, till it is short and tender. Chop the suet very fine, and when the eggs are well beaten together, after the white specks are taken out, pour the liquid over the pounded meat and chopped suet, well kneading together with a clean hand, throwing in the sifted sage, and pepper, and salt, during the operation, so as to let them impregnate the whole mass without being predominant in any part of it. Press the whole, when well mixed, into a wide-mouthed jar, and keep it from the air in a cool place.

They may be made up into small balls, or put into guts, nicely cleaned, when wanting for use. Use very little grease, or lard, in frying them, as they will be almost fat enough to fry themselves without.

TO MAKE FORCE-MEAT BALLS.

Now you are to observe that force-meat balls are a great addition to all made dishes. Made thus :— take three pounds of veal, and a pound of suet, cut fine, and beat in a marble mortar; have a few sweet herbs made fine, a little mace dried and beat fine, and a small nutmeg grated, a little lemon-peel cut very fine, a little pepper and salt, and the yolk of two eggs; mix all these well together, then roll them in little round balls, and some in long balls; roll them in flour, and fry them brown.

COOKING MEAT.

The preparation of meat for the table is usually performed by one of the processes of boiling, roasting or stewing; and much of its excellence as food, or value for the purposes of nutrition, is depending on the manner in which these operations are severally performed.

In boiling meat, particularly that which is salted, if the following particulars are observed, the meat will generally be properly boiled. The water that is used is best if soft; and the meat, after being thoroughly washed, &c., should be placed over the fire in cold water, that the whole may be gradually heated, and thus boiled equally. Salted meat should never be boiled fast; it is better to be simmered only, as fast boiling makes such meat hard. Pieces of meat chosen for boiling, should be of the same thickness throughout, or they will be unequally cooked. An essential condition of boiling meat properly, and have it retain a good appearance, is to keep the pot well skimmed, and steadily but gently boiling. The coagulated albuminous matter that rises on the surface in boiling, if not removed, will attach itself to the meat and injure both its appearance and flavour. Good cooks allow thirty minutes slow boiling to every pound of meat, reckoning from the commencement of the boiling. Flesh or fish boiled in an open vessel, will leave the lean or fibrous part more tender, than if the vessel is left covered. With the farmer, more meat is cooked by boiling than in any other way, and it is, therefore, important that the best and most economical way should always be chosen.

A large part of the meat used in cities is roasted, and every one is aware how much the character of beef or mutton is depending on this operation. With regard to the manner of cooking meat in this way, the taste of no inconsiderable portion of the community appears verging to the Abyssinian standard, and we may soon expect to hear that roasting of beef is entirely dispensed with, and that it is eaten by the ultra fashionables before it has time to cool after being killed. We have some doubts, however, whether man was destined to feed on raw flesh, and believe that the nutritive effect is much increased, and the mechanical labor of the teeth and stomach much diminished, by a proper system of cooking. The true criterion is, that the meat roasted be tender, and this cannot be done by placing it for a few moments before or over a hot fire, by which the outside is burned and the inside left unchanged or raw. The process must be gradual to be complete, and the more perfectly cooked the meat is, the better and more nutritive it will be, and the easier of digestion.

Stewing is nothing else than boiling by means of a small quantity of an aqueous fluid, water or broth, and continuing the operation for a long time to render the substance tender, the texture loose, to make it more sapid, and to retain or concentrate the most valuable parts of animal or vegetable food. The process of stewing must be conducted with a small quantity of water, the heat steady but gentle, so as to raise the fluid only to a simmering heat, and covered so as to prevent the escape of the fluid by evaporation. Much of the good quality of the dishes prepared by stewing, is depending on the management of the fire, for if the heat is too great the softening of the meat will not be as perfect, and water must be frequently added, or it would burn on to the vessel. The kinds of meat most suitable for stewing, or which are the most improved by the process, are those that abound in fibrin or lean, and which are frequently too dry or tough for roasting. In stewing, those portions of meat that cannot be eaten roasted, and are rarely boiled, as the hard muscular or tendinous parts, such as the hocks of beef, are converted into a rich gelatinous nutritive food, of the most savory kind, and can be served up with proper vegetables, or used as gravy or soup. In stewing, the great danger is burning the meat by allowing the water to evaporate. This guarded against, stewed meats are excellent.

FRYING PORK.

Take one fresh egg, beat it, add half a gill of sour

milk, and a sufficient quantity of flour to make a batter; freshen and fry the pork as usual, then dip the pieces in the batter, which will of course adhere; replace them in the fat, and after a little more frying a light and delicate cake will enclose the meat, and thus constitute a dish for a middling sized family, which will tempt the palate of the most fastidious. Try it, ladies.

HOW TO COOK CODFISH.

As Paddy would say, when codfish is boiled it ought not to be boiled at all. It is, however, a little surprising that many a good housewife is not apprised that the dumb or dried codfish ought not to be boiled to have them tender. It operates as an egg, an oyster, or a clam: the more you boil them the harder they get. Over night put the fish to soak in cold water. In the morning it may be removed into a kettle of fresh water, made warm, and set by the fire. Half an hour previous to its being dished up it may be exchanged into a kettle of fresh water, and simmered over the fire nearly to a boiling heat, but no higher. This management does not draw out, but revives and enlivens the nutritious substance in them, and leaves the fish tender and delicious.

CELERY SAUCE FOR ROASTED OR BOILED FOWLS.

Take a large bunch of celery, wash it clean, cut it fine, and boil it slowly in a little water till it is tender; then add a little beaten mace, some nutmeg, pepper, and salt, thickened with a piece of butter rolled in flour. Then boil it up, and pour it in your dish. You may add half a pint of cream, and a glass of white wine.

DIRECTIONS FOR BOILING POTATOES.

Seldom do we see potatoes well cooked, and still more seldom do we see them cooked without waste. Choose your potatoes of an equal size, and put them into a sauce-pan or pot without a lid, with no more water than is sufficient to cover them. More would only spoil them, as the potatoes, on being boiled, yield a considerable portion of water. By being boiled in a vessel without a lid, they do not crack, and all waste is prevented. After the water has come nearly to a boiling, pour it off, and replace the hot by cold water, into which throw a good portion of salt. The cold water sends the heat from the surface to the heart of the potatoe, and makes it mealy. Like all other vegetables they are improved by being boiled with salt. The only proper test of their being done enough is trying them with a fork. When they are boiled, cracking is usually the test of their being done enough; but they will often crack when they are quite raw in the heart. After straining off the water, they should be allowed to stand ten or fifteen minutes on the fire to dry.

ANOTHER.—Select the potatoes designed for dinner a few hours previous; pare them, and throw them into cold water, and let them stand three or four hours; then at a proper time before dinner put them into boiling water, with a handful of salt, and when they have sufficiently boiled turn off the water, leave off the cover, and hang them over the fire to dry. When the steam has passed off, they will then be in the best possible condition for eating. By this method potatoes of even a watery and inferior quality become mealy and good.

WASHING SALADS.

To free salads from insects and worms, they should first be placed in salt water for a few minutes, to kill and bring out the worms, and then washed with fresh water in the usual way. This is an invaluable suggestion, as all salads are subject to insects, and some of them inconceivably small.

IMPROVED METHOD OF MAKING COFFEE.

Put your coffee (after grinding) into a flannel bag, tie it closely, allowing sufficient room to boil freely; put it into the boiler, adding as much water as may be required. After boiling, it will be perfectly clear, without the addition of eggs, &c., having likewise the advantage of retaining its original flavor and strength in greater perfection than when clarified.

TO MAKE GOOD COFFEE OUT OF RYE.

The rye is to be well cleaned, and then boiled till soft, but care is to be taken that it does not burst. It is afterwards to be dried in the sun, or in an oven, and then burnt like coffee, and when ground it is fit for use.

It may be infused and boiled in the usual way; but if coffee equal to Mocha is required, half of this powder mixed with half its weight of real coffee, gives a beverage fit for the Grand Turk, or to be served to the guest at the coffee hamblin of the Palais Royale.

APPLE MOLASSES.

There is many a good housewife who has more faith in her own experience than in the science of chemistry, that knows not the value of apple molasses; but still believes it to be the same kind of tart, smoky, worthless stuff that has from time immemorial been made by boiling down cider. It is not within my province at this time to attempt to convince such that there is a chemical difference, though it might easily be shown that they are almost as different as sugar and vinegar; I would, however, invite them to lay aside their cider this year, and try the plan of boiling down the juice of the apple, that has not been exposed to the air by grinding and pressing. Last autumn I placed a number of bushels of Wetherill's sweeting apples in two large brass kettles, with water just enough to steam them; when they had boiled soft, I turned them into a new splinter basket containing some straw, and placed on them a barrel head, and a heavy weight. The juice was caught in a tub. This was repeated until I had juice enough to fill up the kettles, when I commenced boiling it down, and attended to it strictly, frequently skimming it, till it became of the consistence of cane molasses. The native acids of the fruit imparted a peculiar flavor, otherwise it could hardly be distinguished from the syrup of the cane. It was used in my family for making sweetmeats, for sweetening pies, for dressing on puddings, and griddle cakes, and a variety of other purposes. The cost of making it is very trifling, and the means are within the reach of every farmer.

APPLE BUTTER.

To make this article according to German custom, the host should, in the autumn, invite his neighbors to make up an apple-butter party. Being assembled, let three bushels of fair sweet apples be pared, quartered, and the cores removed: meanwhile let two barrels of clear new cider be boiled down to one half; when this is done commit the prepared apples to the cider, and henceforth let the boiling go on briskly and systematically. But to accomplish the main design, the party must take turns at stirring the contents without cessation, that they do not become attached to the side of the kettle, and be burned. Let this stirring go on till the liquid becomes concrete : in other words, till the amalgamated cider and apples become as thick as hasty pudding; then throw in seasoning of pulverized allspice, when it may be considered as finished and committed to pots for future use. This is apple butter, and will keep sweet for many years.

APPLE JELLY.

Pare, quarter, and core any quantity of fine, sound apples, cover them with water, and boil them till soft; take them out and put them into a sieve, and let all the juice drain from them into the water they were boiled in ; then take the parings and some cores, cover with water and boil them ; then add all the liquor of both together, and boil to a good syrup; then add one pound of sugar to one pint of syrup, and boil fifteen or twenty minutes.

PEACH JELLY.

Wipe the down well off your peaches, which should be free stones, and not too ripe, and cut them in quarters, crack the stones, and break the kernels small; put the peaches and kernels into a covered jar, set them in boiling water, and let them boil till they are soft; strain them through a jelly bag until all the juice is squeezed out : allow a pint of loaf sugar to a pint of juice ; put the sugar and juice into a preserving kettle and boil them twenty minutes, skimming very carefully; put the jelly warm into glasses, and when cold, tie them up with papers wet in French brandy and covered over the top.

NOTE.—Plum and green grape jelly may be made in the same manner with the kernels, which greatly improve the flavor.

CURRANT JELLY [RED OR BLACK].

Strip the fruit in a stone jar, and stew them in a sauce-pan of water, or by boiling it on the hot hearth; strain off the liquor, and to every pint weigh a pound of loaf sugar; put the latter in large lumps into it, in a stone or China vessel, till nearly dissolved; then put it in a preserving pan or kettle, simmer and skim as necessary: when it will jelly on a plate, put it in small glass jars.

RICE JELLY.

This is one of the most nourishing preparations of rice, particularly for valetudinarians or convalescents. It is thus made—Boil a quarter of a pound of rice flour, with half a pound of loaf sugar, in a quart of water, till the whole becomes one glutinous mass; then strain off the jelly, and let it stand to cool. A little of this salubrious food eaten at a time will be found very beneficial to those of a weakly and infirm constitution.

BLACKBERRY CORDIAL.

This syrup is said to be a specific for the summer complaint. From a teaspoonful to a wine-glass according to the age of the patient, must be given at intervals till relieved.

How to make it.—To two quarts of juice of blackberries add one pound of loaf sugar, half an ounce of nutmegs, half an ounce of cinnamon pulverized, one quarter of an ounce of cloves, one quarter of an ounce of allspice, pulverized; boil together for a short time, and when cold add a pint of fourth-proof French brandy.

TO MAKE RASPBERRY JAM.

Take a pint of currant jelly, and a quart of raspberries; bruise them well together, set them over a slow fire, keeping them stirring all the time till it boils; let it boil gently half an hour, and stir it round very often, to keep it from sticking, and rub it through a colander; pour it into your jar, covering it tight: it will keep for a year or two, and have the full flavour of the raspberry.

ORANGE SYRUP.

This syrup, so easily made, can be used so constantly with advantage, that no housekeeper should be without it. Select ripe and thin-skinned fruit, squeeze the juice through a sieve; to every pint add a pound and a half of powdered sugar; boil it slowly, and skim as long as any scum rises; you may then take it off, let it grow cold, and bottle it off. Be sure to secure the corks well. Two tablespoonsful of this syrup, mixed in melted butter, make an admirable sauce for plum or batter pudding; it imparts a fine flavor to custards.

TOMATO CATSUP.

Take a peck of ripe tomatoes (or any other quantity, only observe proportions), mash them well together, and simmer over a slow fire until they are dissolved; strain through a fine sieve; after straining, which requires some pains by mashing and forcing the pulp through the sieve with the hand, add to this liquid pulpy mass half an ounce of cloves, and the same quantity of black pepper grains, one root of garlic, three ounces of horseradish, and a sufficient quantity of salt to make it palatable; boil all these ingredients together over a gradual fire, until you reduce the bulk to one half, then to each quart add two tablespoonsful of vinegar. When it is cool, cork it up in bottles, and in a little time it will be fit for use.

SPICED TOMATOES.

Take a bushel of tomatoes, and pour boiling water over them, skin them, then boil them well, after which add a teaspoonful of salt, a tablespoonful of black pepper, one tablespoonful of Cayenne, half an ounce of cloves, one ounce of mace; mix well, and put the tomatoes in jars, run mutton suet over them, and tie buckskin over the tops: prepared in this way, they will keep a year.

TO PRESERVE TOMATOES IN A FRESH STATE.

The Indiana Farmer says that tomatoes may be kept fresh through the fall and winter, by packing them in jars, laying alternately a layer of dry sand and a layer of tomatoes until the vessel is full; after which cover them up tight to keep the air out, and place them in a dry cellar.

PRESERVATION OF APPLES.

Apples, after remaining as long on the trees as safety from the frost will admit, should be taken directly from the trees, picked carefully by hand, and put into close casks, and kept dry and cool as possible. If suffered to lie on the floor for weeks, they will wither and lose their flavour, without acquiring any additional durability. The best mode of preserving apples for spring use I have found to be putting of them in dry sand as soon as picked. For this purpose dry sand in the heat of summer, and late in October; put down the apples in layers singly, with a covering of sand upon each layer. The singular advantages of this mode of treatment are these: first, the sand keeps the apples from the air, which is essential to their preservation; secondly, the sand checks the evaporation of the apples, thus preserving them in their full flavor, at the same time any moisture yielded by the apples (and some there will be) is absorbed by the sand, so that the apples are kept dry, and all mustiness is prevented. The casks should be headed. Irish potatoes will keep in a good state put up in the same way, and should be put into the barrels as soon as they are dug and gathered.

TO PRESERVE GRAPES AND PLUMS IN A FRESH STATE.

Grapes or plums may be taken from the vines, or trees, and be preserved in a fresh state for use, for a length of time, simply, by alternating them in layers with cotton battings, in a large stone jar, and placing them in a chamber secure from frost. The discovery was accidental. A servant maid in the family of William Mercy, of Union Village, Washington County, about to visit her friends, secured a quantity of plums in this way, to preserve them till her return. They were found to have kept in an excellent condition, long after the fruit had disappeared in the garden. From the hint thus afforded, Mr. Mercy, Mr. Holmes, and one or two neighbours, laid down grapes in this manner last fall, and they enjoyed the luxury of fresh, fine flavored fruit through the winter, until the early part of March.—*Buel's Cultivator.*

PLUMS, PEACHES, TO KEEP FRESH THROUGH THE YEAR.

Beat well up together equal quantities of honey and spring water; pour it into an earthen vessel; put in the fruits all freshly gathered, and cover them quite close. When any of the fruit is taken out, wash it in cold water, and it is fit for immediate use.

TO PRESERVE PUMPKINS IN A FRESH STATE.

Pull them after they have got their growth, and a little before the frost comes on, and put them in a warm dry room. By this method they have been kept in a dry state for two years.

TO PRESERVE GREEN CORN FOR BOILING.

Pluck the corn when fit for eating; strip down the husk so as to remove the silk, and then replace it. Pack it away in a barrel, and pour on strong pickle, such as is used for meat, with a weight to keep it down, and you will have a good sea stock parboiled, and then boiled to make it perfectly fresh and sweet as when taken from the stock.—*Genesee Farmer.*

PRESERVATION OF CABBAGE.

After they have got their growth, and are gathered in the fall, cut off their loose leaves and stalks, that nothing remains but the sound part of the head: they may be headed up in a tight cask. By thus excluding them from the air they may be kept for a long time. Those intended for the longest keeping should be put into small casks, as they will soon spoil when exposed to the air.

TO PRESERVE GREEN PEAS.

Gather them while they are yet tender; shell and dry them. If they can be dried in the shade without moulding so much the better. Take them the following winter, and after soaking them in warm water over night you will find them the next day swollen to the size, and being as green and tender as they were when gathered. Then boil them as usual, and you will have green peas in midwinter. Don't let them get too old and hard before they are gathered.

FROZEN POTATOES.

In the time of frost the only precaution necessary is to retain the potatoes in a perfectly dark place for some days after a thaw has commenced. In America, where they are sometimes frozen as hard as stones, they rot if thawed in open day; but if thawed in darkness they do not rot, and lose very little of their natural odour and properties.

TO DRY CHERRIES.

To every five pounds of cherries, stoned, weigh one of sugar double refined, put the fruit into a preserving kettle with very little water, make both scalding hot; take the fruit out and immediately dry them; put them into a kettle again, stirring the sugar between each layer of cherries; let it stand to melt, then set the kettle on the fire, and make it scalding hot as before, take it off, and repeat this thrice with the sugar; drain them from the syrup, and lay them singly to dry on dishes in the sun, or on the stove. When dry put them into a sieve, dip it into a pan of cold water, and draw it instantly out again, and pour them on a fine soft cloth; dry them, and set them once more in the hot sun, or on a stove; keep them in a box, with layers of white paper, in a dry place. This way is the best to give plumpness to the fruit, as well as colour and flavour.

DRIED APPLES AND PEARS.

The apples and pears which arrive here in a dried state from France are thus prepared :—The fruit is put into boiling water, in which it is left until it becomes soft. It is then taken out and carefully peeled. The stem being left on to prevent any loss of juices, it is placed on a strainer, under which is a dish; when peeled it is put into an oven heated to the ordinary temperature for bread, and left there twenty-four hours. When taken out and cold, the fruit is pressed flat, and after being plunged into its own juice, which has been set apart for that purpose, it is packed in boxes and exported. For family use it might be packed away in stone jars.

DRIED PEACHES.

Just before fully ripe, peel peaches, either plum or soft peaches, take out the nuts, put them in boiling water till they are a little soft; take them out, and throw them into a pailful of cold water; when cold, drain and weigh them. To every pound of peaches put half a pound of powdered loaf sugar. Lay the peaches in a kettle and sprinkle the sugar until it is all in. Let it remain until the syrup runs sufficiently to allow putting it on over a very slow fire when the sugar is all melted. Let them boil slowly till the peaches look clear; then put them in a large bowl, and let them remain all night. The next morning place them snugly in dishes, and put them into the sun to dry. Turn them over every day until they are sufficiently dry to be packed in boxes or in jars. The soft peaches are as good, if not better than the plum, and the nut is taken out much easier. The peaches will break some of them in doing. After they have been in the sun two or three days, with a teaspoon and a silver fork draw the broken pieces together in the form and size of a peach, and they will dry solid. There will be more syrup than can be dried with them, which may be used by boiling some peaches prepared as above in the spare syrup. These will be inferior, but still good.

TO MAKE PEACH SWEETMEATS.

To one pound of peaches put half a pound of good brown sugar, with half a pint of water to dissolve it, first clarifying it with an egg; then boil the peaches and sugar together, skimming the egg off, which will rise on the top till it is the thickness of a jelly. If you wish to do them whole, do not peel them, but put them into boiling water and give them a boil. Then take them out, and wipe them dry. Pears are done in the same way.

MAKING BRANDY PEACHES.

Scald them in hot water, then dip them in strong hot ley, rub them with a cloth, and throw them into cold water; make a syrup of three-quarters of a pound of sugar to one pound of fruit, and when cold put an equal quantity of brandy.

TO PRESERVE QUINCES WHOLE.

Take the weight of your quinces in sugar, and put a pint of water to a pound of sugar; make it into a syrup, and clarify it; then core your quinces, and pare them, and put them into your syrup, and let it boil till it be all clear; then put in three spoonsful of jelly, which must be made thus :—Over night lay your quince kernels in water; then strain them, and put them into your quinces, and let them have but one boil afterward.

TO PRESERVE STRAWBERRIES WHOLE.

Take equal weights of the fruit and double refined loaf sugar; lay the former in a large dish, and sprinkle half the sugar in fine powder over; give a gentle shake to the dish, that the sugar may touch the under sides of the fruit. Next day make a thin syrup with the remainder of the sugar, and instead of water allow one pint of red currant juice to every pound of strawberries. In this simmer them until sufficiently jellied.

TO PRESERVE STRAWBERRIES IN WINE.

Put a quantity of the finest large strawberries into a large gooseberry bottle, and strew in three large spoonsful of sugar. Fill up with moderate wine or fine sherry.

TO PRESERVE RASPBERRIES.

Pick your raspberries in a dry day, just before they are fully ripe; lay them in a dish; beat and sift their weight of fine sugar, and strew it over them. To every quart of raspberries take a quart of red currant jelly, and put to its weight of fine sugar; boil and skim it well. Then put in your raspberries, and give them a scald. Take them off, and let them stand two hours. Then set them on again, and scald until they look clear.

TO PRESERVE GREEN FIGS.

The figs may be gathered when they have got their growth, and when they begin to turn to be ripe. Put them in a sieve, and pour boiling water over them to stand about an hour, then weigh the sugar and allow pound for pound, put them in a kettle and boil with the syrup, then take them out, and put them into dishes in the sun, boil the syrup down, put the figs back, and let them boil a short time.

TOMATO FIGS.

Take six pounds of sugar to one peck or sixteen pounds of the fruit. Scald and remove the skin in the usual way. Cook them over a fire, their own juice being sufficient without the addition of water, until the sugar penetrates and they are clarified. They are then taken out, spread on dishes, flattened and dried in the sun. A small quantity of the syrup should be occasionally sprinkled over them whilst drying; after which pack them down in boxes, treating each layer with powdered sugar. The syrup is afterwards concentrated and bottled for use. They keep well from year to year, and retain surprisingly their flavor, which is nearly that of the best quality of fresh figs! The pear-shaped or single tomatoes answer the purpose best. Ordinary brown sugar may be used, a large portion of which is retained in the syrup.

TO PRESERVE CITRON WATERMELON.

Pare the dark green from the outside, and scrape the soft pulp from the inside of the melon; cut in slices, boil it in alum water till clear. Throw it into spring water, where it may lie two or three hours, changing the water frequently. To one pound of fruit take one pound of sugar. Make a syrup of half the quantity of sugar, and boil with it all the melon until done, when it will be transparent. At the expiration of two or three days take the jelly from it, and add the remaining half of sugar. Boil and pour it over the melon, which will be ready for use. Season it with ginger.

Some persons follow the above receipt, scalding the melons in alum water; others soak them in pure water, and scald them by turning on the boiling syrup. If this method does not soften them enough, they should be scalded in the syrup; for as they are very hard, they should be well softened by heat. Another method is to scald them in salt water till they are soft. Then put them into spring water as directed in the above receipt, and change the water till they are sufficiently fresh. When the melons are prepared by either of those ways, then dissolve the sugar in water, using no more water than is necessary to dissolve it, and turn it, scalding hot, on the melons, and let it remain a few days, and then it will have become thin from the juice of the melons, and it should be again boiled awhile and reduced to a greater degree of consistence, and then pour on the melons. It may be necessary to boil it the third time.

TO PRESERVE GOLDEN PIPPINS.

Take the rind of an orange, boil it very tender, and lay it in cold water for three days; take two dozen golden pippins, pare one quarter of them, and boil them to a strong jelly, and run it through a jelly-bag till it is clear; take the same quantity, pare them, and take out the cores; put three pounds of loaf sugar in a preserving kettle, with three half pints of spring water. When it boils, skim it well, and put in your pippins, with the orange rind, cut in long thin slips; let them boil fast till the sugar is thick, and it will almost candy. Then put in three half-pints of pippin-jelly, and boil it fast till the jelly is clear. Then squeeze in the juice of a lemon, give it a boil, and put them in glass jars with the orange-peel.

TO PRESERVE GRAPES.

Get some fine grapes, not over ripe, either red or white, and pick out all the speckled ones. Put them in a jar, with a quarter of a pound of sugar-candy, and fill the jar with French brandy. Tie them down close, and keep them in a dry place.

TO PRESERVE CRAB APPLES.

Wash your fruit; cover the bottom of your preserving-kettle with grape leaves; put in the apples; hang them over the fire, with a very little water, and cover them closely. Do not allow them to boil, but let them simmer gently till they are yellow. Take them out, and spread them on a large dish to cool; pare and core them; put them again into the kettle, with fresh vine-leaves under and over them, and a very little water; hang them over the fire till they are green, but do not let them boil; take them out, weigh them, and allow a pound of loaf sugar to a pound of crab apples; put to the sugar just water enough to dissolve; when it is all melted, put it on the fire, and boil the apples till they are quite clear and soft. Put them in jars, and pour the warm liquor over them. When cold, tie them up with brandy paper.

TO PRESERVE CRANBERRIES.

Wash your cranberries, weigh them, and to each pound allow a pound of loaf sugar; dissolve the sugar in a very little water (about half a pint of water to a pound of sugar), and set it on the fire in a preserving-kettle; boil it near ten minutes, skimming it well; then put in your cranberries, and boil them slowly till they are quite soft, and of a fine colour.

Put them warm into your jars or glasses, and tie them up with brandy paper when cold; when opened for use they should be tied up again immediately, as exposure to the air spoils them.

PRESERVED PINEAPPLE.

Pare your pineapples, and cut them in thin round slices; weigh the slices, and to each pound allow a pound of loaf sugar; dissolve the sugar in a very small quantity of water, stir it, and set it over the fire in a preserving kettle; boil it ten minutes, skimming it well; then put in it the pineapple slices, and boil them till they are clear and soft, but not till they break—about half an hour, or perhaps less time, will suffice. Let them cool in a large dish or pan before you put them into your jars, which you must do carefully, lest they break. Pour the syrup over them, and tie them up with brandy paper.

TO CLARIFY SUGAR FOR PRESERVES.

Break as much as is required in large lumps, and put a pound to a half-pint of water in a bowl, and it will dissolve better than when broken small. Set it over the fire, and add the white of an egg well beat; let it boil up, and when ready to run over, pour a little cold water in it to give it a check; but when it rises the second time, take it off the fire, and set it by in the pan a quarter of an hour, during which the foulness will sink to the bottom, and leave a black scum on the top, which take off gently with a skimmer, and pour the syrup into a vessel very quickly from the sediment.

TO PICKLE OYSTERS.

Put the oysters on the fire, and let them simmer

till the gills begin to shrivel, then take them up and wipe them carefully in a towel; strain the liquor, and put it on to boil, with a little salt, whole pepper, and mace; when well boiled, to a quart of liquor add one half pint of Madeira wine, and the same quantity of good vinegar; the liquor must be nearly cold before it is poured on the oysters.

TO PICKLE WALNUTS.

Scald slightly, and rub off the first skin of one hundred walnuts, before they have a hard shell. This may be easily ascertained by trying them with a pin. Put them in a strong cold brine, put new brine the third and sixth days, and take them out and dry them on the ninth. Take an ounce of each—of long pepper-pods, black pepper, ginger, and allspice, a quarter of an ounce of cloves, some blades of mace, and a tablespoonful of white mustard-seed; bruise the whole together. Put into a jar a layer of walnuts, strew them well over with the mixture, and proceed in the same manner till all are covered; then boil three quarts of good vinegar with sliced horse-radish and ginger, pour it hot over, which may be repeated for three or four days, always keeping the pickles closely covered; add at the last boiling a few cloves of garlic, or shalots. In five months they will be fit for use.

TO PICKLE CUCUMBERS.

Select a sufficient quantity of the size you prefer, which probably cannot be done at one time. Put them in a stone pot, and pour over them a strong brine; to this add a small bit of alum, to secure the colour. Let them stand a week; then exchange the brine for clear water, in which they must remain two or three days. Boil the best northern cider vinegar, and, when nearly cool, pour it over the cucumbers, having previously turned off the water. Prepared in this manner, with the addition of cloves, allspice, mustard, and cinnamon, boiled in the vinegar, pickles of every kind will keep for a year. In pickling cauliflowers, tomatoes, and other vegetables which easily absorb the vinegar—the spiced vinegar should be added when cold.

ANOTHER.—To each hundred of cucumbers put a pint of salt, and pour on boiling water sufficient to cover the whole; cover them tight to prevent the steam from escaping, and in this condition let them stand for twenty-four hours; they are then to be taken out; and after being wiped perfectly dry, care being taken that the skin is not broken, place them in the jar in which they are to be kept. Boiling vinegar (if spice be used, it should be boiled with the vinegar) is then to be put to them, the jar closed tight; and in a fortnight delicious pickles are produced, as green as when they were on the vines.

ANOTHER, WITH WHISKEY AND VINEGAR.—Sir:—From the scarcity of vinegar last season, I was led to make trial of a mode of preserving, or pickling cucumbers, that I should not have attempted under other circumstances. But it has succeeded so well with me that I am desirous other housewives should partake of the benefit. I gathered the cucumbers from the vines, and without any other preparation than washing them clean, dropped them into a stone jar containing a mixture of whiskey and water—one part of the former to three of the latter. I secured them against gnats, flies, and external air, by tying a flannel close over the top, and laying over this a board and stone. I neither moved nor examined them until Christmas, when I found them not merely equal, but decidedly superior to any pickles I had ever tasted. They were hard and of a fine flavor, and, what has been particularly admired in them, they retained the original color of the cucumber, not exhibiting the green, poisonous appearance of pickles that had been salted and scalded in copper. My whiskey and water (no salt having been used or heat employed) was now excellent vinegar for the table.

TO PICKLE CABBAGE.

Slice the cabbage crosswise; put it on an earthen dish, and sprinkle a handful of salt over it; cover it with another dish, and let it stand twenty-four hours; put it in a colander to drain, and lay it in a jar; take white wine vinegar enough to cover it, a little cloves, mace, and allspice. Put them in whole; boil it up, and put it over hot or cold, which you like best, and cover it close with a cloth. Then tie it over with leather.

TO PICKLE TOMATOES.

Gather the tomatoes when they are turning to be ripe. Put them in layers in a jar with garlic, mustard seed, horse-radish, spices as you like, filling up the jar, occasionally putting a little fine salt proportionably to the quantity laid down, and which is intended to preserve the tomatoes. When the jar is full, pour on cold, good cider vinegar till all is covered; then cork up tight.

TO PICKLE ONIONS.

Take onions when they are dry enough to lay up

for winter, not too large; put them in a pot, and cover with spring water, with a handful of salt. Let them boil up; then strain them off, and take the coats off; wipe them dry, and put them in glass jars, with some blades of mace and cloves, and a nutmeg cut fine. Take good vinegar; boil it up with a little salt, and put it over the onions. When they are cold cork them close, and tie a bladder, or leather over it.

TO PICKLE BEETS.

Boil your beets, then peel and cut them, and put them in a jar. Take as much vinegar as will cover them; boil it and add thereto half an ounce of whole pepper, half an ounce of allspice, a little ginger, and one head of garlic (say to one gallon of vinegar). When the vinegar is cold put it over them, and in two days they will be fit for use.

TO PICKLE MELON MANGOES.

Take as many green melons as you want, and slit them two-thirds up the middle, and with a spoon take all the seeds out; put them in strong spring water and salt for twenty-four hours. Then drain them in a sieve. Mix half a pound of white mustard, two ounces of long pepper, the same of allspice, half an ounce of cloves and mace, a good quantity of garlic and horse-radish cut in slices, and a quarter of an ounce of cayenne pepper. Fill the insides full of this mixture; put a small skewer through the end, and tie it around with packthread close to the skewer; put them in a jar, and boil up vinegar, with some of the mixture in it, and pour over the melons; cover them down close, and let them stand twenty-four hours. Then put them in your kettle, and simmer over the fire till they are green. You may do large cucumbers the same way.

TO PICKLE GHERKINS.

Take five hundred gherkins, and have ready a large earthen pan of spring water and salt; to every gallon of water add two pounds of salt; mix it well together, and throw in your gherkins; wash them out in two hours, and put them to drain; let them drain very dry, and put them in a jar; take a gallon of good vinegar, and put into a bell-metal kettle, and add half an ounce of cloves and mace, an ounce of allspice, one ounce of white mustard seed, a stick of horse-radish cut into slices, six bay leaves, two or three races of ginger cut fine, a nutmeg cut fine, and a handful of salt; boil it up in the kettle all together, and put it over the gherkins; cover them close down, and let them stand twenty-four hours, then put them in your kettle and simmer over the fire till they are green: be careful not to let them boil, if you do, it will spoil them; then put them in your jar, and cover them down close till cold; then tie them over with a bladder, and a leather over that; put them in a cold, dry place. Mind always to keep your pickles tied down close, and take them out with a wooden spoon.

TO PICKLE GRAPES.

Take grapes at the full growth, but not ripe; cut them in small bunches, put them in a stone jar, with vine leaves between every layer of grapes; then take as much spring water as you think will cover them, put in a pound of bay salt, and as much white salt as will make it bear an egg; dry your bay salt and pound it, it will melt the sooner; put it into a copper or bell-metal kettle, boil it, and skim well as it boils, take all the black scum off, but not the white scum: when it has boiled a quarter of an hour, let it stand to cool and settle;

when it is almost cold pour the clear liquor on the grapes, lay vine leaves on the top, tie them down close with a linen cloth, cover them over with another, let them be dried between the cloths; then take two quarts of vinegar, one quart of spring water, and one pound of sugar, let it boil a little while, skim it as it boils, very clean, let it stand till it is quite cold, dry your jar with a cloth, put fresh vine leaves at the bottom, and between every layer of grapes, and on the top; then pour the clear pickle on the grapes, fill your jar that the pickle may be above the grapes; tie a thin piece of board in a piece of flannel, lay it on the top of the jar to keep the grapes under the pickle; tie them up with a bladder, and then a leather.

TO PICKLE PEACHES.

Take your peaches when they are at their full growth, just before they begin to turn ripe; be sure they are not bruised; then take spring water as much as you think will cover them, make it salt enough to bear an egg, then put in your peaches, and lay a thin board over them, to keep them under the water; let them stand three days, and then take them out and wipe them very carefully with a fine soft cloth, and lay them in your glass jar; then take as much good vinegar as will fill the jar; to every gallon put two or three heads of garlic, a good deal of ginger cut fine, half an ounce of cloves, mace, and nutmeg; mix your pickle well together, and pour over your peaches: tie them close with a bladder and leather, and they will be fit for use in three months. You may pickle nectarines and apricots the same way.

TO PICKLE SOUR KROUT.

Chop the heads of large cabbages very fine, and

strew it in layers in a barrel, with alternately a handful of salt, mixed with a few caraway seeds, till the barrel is filled. A heavy weight is next to be placed on the mass, and a fermentation soon commences. After this has subsided, the weight is removed, and the barrel is headed for use. This preparation is highly relished by those accustomed to it, when boiled with beef.

TO MAKE CURRANT WINE.

To each gallon of currant juice, add two gallons of water, and to each gallon of the mixture, add three and a half pounds of good brown sugar, and put into good barrels. After it has done fermenting, it should be bunged tight for two or three weeks; then it should be racked off, and put into clean strong casks. If you wish to give it more body, add to each barrel, after it has been racked off, one gallon of good French brandy. Gooseberry wine may be made in the same manner.

PARSNIP WINE.

Wine made of parsnip-root approaches nearer to the Malmsley of Madeira and Canaries than any other wine; (as we learn from our friend " the Doctor;") it is made with little expense or trouble, and only requires to be kept a few years to make it agreeable to the palate as it is wholesome to the body. To every four pounds of parsnips, clean and quartered, put one gallon of water: boil them till they are quite tender; drain them through a sieve, but do not bruise them, as no remedy would clear them afterwards. Pour the liquor into a tub, and to each gallon add three pounds of loaf sugar, and half an ounce of crude tartar. When cooled to the temperature of 75 degrees, put in a little new yeast; let it stand four days in a warm room, then turn it. The mixture should, if possible, be fermented in a temperature of 60 degrees. September and March are the best seasons for making the wine. When the fermentation has subsided, bung down the cask and let the wine stand at least twelve months before bottling.

GINGER WINE.

Of bruised ginger twelve pounds, water ten gallons. Boil for half an hour; add twenty-eight pounds of sugar; boil till dissolved; then cool, and put the liquor along with fourteen lemons sliced and three pints of good French brandy; add a little yeast, and ferment; bung it up for three months, and then bottle it.

ORANGE WINE.

Of sugar twenty-three pounds, water ten gallons; boil, and clarify with the white of six eggs; pour the boiling liquor upon the parings of one hundred oranges; add the strained juice of these oranges and half a pint of good fresh yeast; let it work for three or four days; then strain it into a barrel; bung it up loosely. In a month add half a gallon of good French brandy, and in three months it will be fit to drink. Wines may also be made of blackberries and other English fruits, upon the same principles. The above are the methods generally employed; but most persons have peculiar ways of proceeding, which may indeed be varied to infinity, and so to produce at pleasure a sweet or dry wine, the sweet not being so thoroughly fermented as the dry. The addition of brandy destroys the flavour of the wine, and it is better to omit it entirely (except for elder or port wine, whose flavour is so strong that it cannot well be injured), and to increase the strength by augmenting the quantity of raisins or sugar. In general, the must for wines ought to be made of six pounds of raisins, or four pounds of sugar to the gallon, allowing for that contained in the fruit.

TO MAKE METHEGLIN.

Of honey fifty weight, boiling water a sufficient quantity to fill a thirty-two gallon cask; stir it well for a day or two; add yeast, and ferment. Some boil the honey in the water for an hour or two, but this hinders its due fermentation.

TO MAKE MEAD.

Take ten gallons of water, two gallons of honey, and a handful of raced ginger; then take two lemons, cut them in pieces, and put them into it; boil it very well; keep skimming it; let it stand all night in the same vessel you boil it in. The next morning barrel it up with two or three spoonsful of good yeast. In two or three weeks after you may bottle it.

TO MAKE HOP BEER.

For half a barrel of beer, take half a pound of hops and half a gallon of molasses. Boil the hops, adding to them a teacupful of powdered ginger, in about a pailful and a half of water, that is, a quantity sufficient to extract the virtue of the hops. When sufficiently boiled or brewed, take it up, and strain it through a sieve, into a tub; add the molasses, shaking or stirring it well with a wooden ladle, that it may be thoroughly mixed. Then put it into your barrel, and fill up with water quite to the bung, observing to shake the barrel well afterwards; the bung must be left open to allow it to work. You must be careful to keep it constantly filled up with water whenever it works over. When sufficiently worked it may be bottled, adding a spoonful of molasses to each bottle.

TO MAKE SPRUCE BEER.

Put four gallons of cold water into a keg with one head out; then boiling four gallons more, put that in also; add two quarts of molasses, or sweeten to your taste, and one large wine glass of the essence of spruce, observing to stir them well together for several minutes. When about blood warm, add one pint of good yeast, the whole being well stirred together. The top should be covered with the head, and set up carefully to work, and in two days it will be fit to bottle. By packing the bottles away in sand in the cellar, or a cool place, they will be kept from bursting, and in two or three days it will be ripe for drinking.

NOTE.—By boiling about a pint of hops in the winter, observing to strain it all through a sieve when putting it into the keg, it will keep good for a long time.

ANOTHER METHOD OF MAKING GOOD BEER.—Put two quarts of molasses into a keg, with eight gallons of cold water, and stir it well, and leave one head out. Boil two ounces allspice, two ounces ginger, two ounces hops, and half-a-pint of Indian meal, in four quarts of water, about an hour; strain it into the keg while hot, stirring it all well together, and in twenty-four hours it will be fit for use, or to bottle.

TAR BEER FOR CONSUMPTION.

The following has been handed to the Philadelphia Inquirer for insertion, as a valuable and efficacious remedy in consumption:

Three quarts of pure water,
One quart of wheat bran,
One pint of tar,
Half-a-pint of honey.

Let them simmer over a slow fire, for three hours, in a new stone vessel; when cool, add half a pint of brewer's yeast; let it stand thirty-six hours, and it is fit for use; it must be kept in a cool place. Take a wine-glass full before each meal.

TO MAKE PERSIMMON BEER.

Take two-thirds persimmons, and one third corn-meal. Mix them well together, and bake in loaves, till they are firm and hard; they should bake slow, taking care not to burn them. Then take the loaves and throw in a clean tub, and pour on warm water enough to soften them; when all is mashed up, it will be a thin dough. Then add as much boiling water as there is dough; after stirring it sufficiently strain it through a sieve, and put it into a keg or barrel, and in a day or two it will be fit for use.

ATTAR OF ROSES.

The Royal Society of Edinburgh received from Dr. Monroe the following account of the manner in which this costly perfume is prepared in the East. Steep a large quantity of the petals of roses, freed from every extraneous matter, in pure water, in an earthen or wooden vessel, which is exposed daily to the sun, and housed at night, till a scum rises to the surface. This is the attar, which is carefully absorbed by a very small piece of cotton tied to the end of a stick. The oil collected, squeeze out of the cotton into a phial, stop it for use. The collection of it should be continued whilst any scum is produced.

MODE OF REFINING WINE AND CIDER.

Take new sweet skim-milk drawn at night and skimmed the following morning, or morning's milk, skimmed at night, one pint to a quarter cask; pour it into the liquor to be refined, the coldest weather in the winter, and stir it up thoroughly to incorporate it completely, let it settle, and your work is done. The liquor will be pure and fine, and will have a peculiar richness imparted to it by the process.

TO MAKE VINEGAR.

Get a good cask and put it in your cellar. Procure a gallon of good vinegar, and let it stand in your cask a day or two, occasionally shaking it around the cask. You may then commence filling up your cask gradually with whiskey and water, in the proportion of one gallon of the former to eight of the latter. It is best not to fill up too fast at first; but wait a week or two before you add again. By this process you may always keep an abundant supply of the purest vinegar.

SODA FOR WASHING.

To five gallons of water add a pint-and-a-half of soft or hard soap, and two ounces sub-carbonate of soda; put the clothes (after soaking over night) into the mixture when at boiling heat, rubbing the parts most soiled with soap. Boil them one hour, drain, rub, and rinse them in warm water: after being put into indigo water, they are fit for drying. Half the soap, and more than half the labor, is saved by washing in this manner.

HOW TO MAKE STARCH.

To make starch from wheat, the grain is steeped

in cold water until it becomes soft and yields a milky juice by pressure; it is then put into sacks of linen, and pressed in a vat filled with cold water ; as long as any milky juice exudes the pressure is continued. The fluid gradually becomes clear, and a white powder subsides, which is starch.

PRESERVING MILK.

A foreign journal states, that some milk was lately exhibited in Liverpool from on board a Swedish vessel, that was several months old, having made two voyages from Sweden to the West Indies and back again, and remained perfectly sweet aad fresh. The manner of preparing it is as follows :—

The bottles are made clean and sweet, and the milk is milked directly into them, without the intervention of a pail. As fast as they are filled they are closely corked, and the corks wired down as in bottling cider. The bottles are placed, when filled, in a boiler, a layer of straw and a layer of bottles, until the layer is full. Fill the boiler with cold water, kindle a fire, and let it heat gradually ; when it begins to boil withdraw the fire, and let the bottles remain till cold. They must then be taken out, packed in hampers, with straw or sawdust, and stowed in the coolest part of the ship. The milk so exhibited was above eighteen months old, and was of excellent quality. It is evident this discovery will be the most available at sea; but where bottles could be easily obtained, many families living in cities and villages who keep a cow, might, by preserving some in this way, furnish themselves with a supply for the time a cow usually goes dry during the winter. In any event the experiment could cost but little.

SUBSTITUTE FOR CREAM.

Beat up the whole of a fresh egg in a basin, and then pour boiling tea or water over it gradually, to prevent it curdling. In flavour and richness this preparation resembles cream.

PRESERVATION OF EGGS.

Relative to the preservation of eggs by immersion in lime-water, Mr Peschier has given most satisfactory evidence of the efficacy of the process. Eggs, which he had preserved for six years in this way, being boiled and tried, were found perfectly fresh and good; and a confectioner of Geneva has used a whole cask preserved by the same means. In a small way eggs may be thus preserved in jars, or other vessels. They are to be introduced when quite fresh, the jar filled after the eggs are put in with lime water, a little powdered lime sprinkled in at last, and t en the jar closely corked. To prepare the lime-water, twenty or thirty pints of water are to be mixed up with five or six pounds of slacked quick lime put into a covered vessel, allowed to clear by standing, and the lime-water immediately used.

ANOTHER.—Eggs may, with proper care, be kept perfectly fresh, not only through the winter, but almost any length of time. The care necessary for this purpose is to render the shell impervious to the air ; or to place them in such a situation that the yolk may not come directly in contact with the shell but remain surrounded by the albumen or white, which is known to withstand the effects of the air much longer without alteration than the yolk. The eggs should be placed in a keg, on the small end ; and every layer should be filled in with salt or sand, to keep them in that position. If they are wanted to be kept for any length of time, there should be a good coat on the top, and the keg headed up. And it would be a great improvement to immerse the eggs previous to their being packed, in a mixture of lard or tallow and beeswax, with an addition of a small quantity of resin, to render the mixture more adhesive. Eggs thus prepared and packed, which might be done at a trifling expense, would continue good for a year or more.

ANOTHER.—One bushel of quick lime, thirty-two ounces of salt, eight ounces of cream of tartar. Mix the whole together, with as much water as will reduce the composition to such a consistency that an egg, when put into it, will swim. Then pack the eggs into jars, or kegs, and pour on the liquid till they are covered.

RECEIPTS FOR HOUSEKEEPERS.

Those who make candles will find it a great improvement to steep the wicks in lime water and saltpetre, and dry them. The flame is clearer, and the tallow will not run.

Britannia ware should be first rubbed gently with a woollen cloth and sweet oil; then washed in warm suds, and rubbed with soft leather and whiting. Thus treated it will retain its beauty to the last.

New iron should be very gradually heated at first. After it has become inured to the heat it is not as likely to crack.

It is a good plan to put new earthenware into cold water, and let it heat gradually until it boils, then cool again. Brown earthenware, in particular, may be toughened in this way. A handful of rye, or wheat bran, thrown in while it is boiling, will preserve the glazing, so that it will not be destroyed by acid or salt.

Clean a brass kettle before using it for cooking, with salt and vinegar.

The oftener carpets are shaken the longer they will wear. The dirt that collects under them grinds out the thread.

If you wish to preserve fine teeth, always clean them thoroughly after you have eaten your last meal at night.

Do not wrap knives and forks in woollens; wrap them in good strong paper. Steel is injured by lying in woollen.

Suet keeps good all the year round, if chopped and packed down in a stone jar, covered with molasses.

Barley straw is the best for beds. Dry corn husks slit in shreds are better than straw.

Brass and irons should be cleaned, done up in papers, and put in a dry place during summer.

When molasses is used for cooking, it is a prodigious improvement to boil and skim it before you use it. It takes out the unpleasant raw taste, and makes it almost as good as sugar. Where molasses is used much for cooking, it is well to prepare one or two gallons in this way at a time.

Never allow ashes to be taken up in wood, or put into wood. Always have your tinder box and lamp ready for use in case of sudden alarm. Have important papers all together, where you can lay your hands on them at once in case of fire.

Use hard soap to wash your clothes, and soft to wash your floor. Soft soap is so slippery that it wastes a good deal in washing clothes.

It is easy to have a supply of horse radish all winter. Have a quantity grated while the root is in perfection, put it in bottles, fill it with vinegar, and keep it corked tight.

Woollen goods should be washed in very hot water with soap, and as soon as the article is cleansed, immerse it in cold water, let it then be wrung and hung up to dry.

INDIAN POUND CAKE.

Eight eggs; the weight of eight eggs in powdered sugar; the weight of six eggs in Indian meal, sifted; half a pound of butter; one nutmeg, grated, or a teaspoonful of cinnamon; stir the butter and sugar to a cream; beat the eggs very light; stir the meal and eggs, alternately, into the butter and sugar; grate in the nutmeg, stir all well. Butter a tin pan, put in the mixture, and bake it in a moderate oven.

CUP CAKE.

Five eggs, two large teacupsful of molasses, the same of brown sugar, rolled fine; the same of fresh butter, one cup of rich milk, five cups of flour, sifted, half a cup of powdered allspice and cloves, half a cup of ginger, cut up the butter in the milk, and warm them slightly; warm also the molasses, and stir it into the milk and butter; then stir in, gradually, the sugar, and set it away to get cool. Beat the eggs very light, and stir them into the mixture alternately with the flour, add the ginger and other spice, and stir the whole very hard. Butter small tins, nearly fill them with the mixture, and bake the cake in a moderate oven.

MILK BISCUIT.

Two pounds of flour, sifted, half a pound of butter,

two eggs, six wine-glasses of milk, two wine-glasses of the best brewer's yeast, or three of good homemade yeast; cut the butter into the milk, and warm it slightly on the top of the stove, or near the fire; sift the flour into a pan, and pour the milk and butter into it, beat the eggs, and pour them in also, lastly the yeast, mix all well together with a knife; flour your paste board, put the lump of dough on it, and knead it very hard. Then cut your dough in small pieces, and knead them into round balls, stick the tops of them with a fork. Lay them in buttered pans and set them to rise. They will probably be light in an hour; when they are quite light, put them in a moderate oven to bake.

BUTTER BISCUITS.

Half a pound of butter, two pounds of flour sifted, half a pint of milk, or cold water, a teaspoonful of salt; cut up the butter in the flour, and put the salt to it, wet it to a stiff dough with the milk, or water; mix it well with a knife, throw some flour on the paste board, take the dough out of the pan, and knead it very well. Roll it out into a large thick sheet, and beat it very hard on both sides with the rolling-pin; beat it a long time, cut it out with a tin, or cup, into small round thick cakes. Beat each cake on both sides, with a rolling-pin, prick them with a fork, put them in buttered pans, and bake them of a light brown in a slow oven.

SPONGE CAKE, CALLED IN FRANCE BISCUIT.

Take ten eggs, and beat them till very thick and smooth, add gradually a pound of powdered loaf-sugar, rub a lump of loaf-sugar all over the rind of a large lemon, to draw the juice to the surface; then grate the peel of the lemon, and stir it into the mixture, together with the lump of sugar. Squeeze in the juice of the lemon, and add two tablespoonsful of rose water. Beat the mixture very hard; then take half a pound of potatoe flour (which is best), or else of fine wheat flour, and stir it in very lightly and slowly. It must be baked immediately.

Have ready some small square or oblong cases of thick white paper, with an edge turned up all around, and sewed at the corners. They should be about a finger in length, half a finger in breadth, and an inch and a half in depth. Either butter these paper-cases, or sift white sugar all over the inside, put some of the mixture in each case, but do not fill them to the top, grate loaf sugar over the top of each, and bake them quickly.

These cakes are much better when baked in paper cases, tins being generally too thick for them; no cake requires greater care in baking. If the oven is not hot enough, both at top and bottom, they will fall and be heavy, and lose their shape.

RICE CAKE.

Take half a pound of rice and wash it well, put it into a pint of cream, or milk, and boil it soft; let it get cold, then stir into it alternately a quarter of a pound of sugar, two ounces of butter, eight eggs, well beaten (having left out the whites of four), and a wine-glass of rose water, or else the grated peel of a lemon. Mix all well, butter a mould or a deep pan with straight sides, and spread grated bread crumbs all over its inside. Put in the mixture, and bake it three-quarters of an hour. Ground rice is the best for this cake. If any of the cake is left, you may next day cut it into slices, and fry them in butter.

Or, instead of baking the mixture in a large cake, you may put flour on your hands, and roll it into balls. Make a batter of beaten eggs, sugar, and grated bread, dip the balls into it, and fry them in butter.

POTATOE CAKE.

Roast in the ashes a dozen small or six large potatoes. When done, peel them, and put them into a pan with a little salt, and the rind of a lemon grated. Add a quarter of a pound of butter, or half a pint of cream, and a quarter of a pound of sugar. Having mashed the potatoes with this mixture, rub it through a colander, and stir it very hard; then set it away to cool. Beat eight eggs, and stir them gradually into the mixture. Season it with a teaspoonful of mixed spice, and half a glass of rosewater; butter a mould or a deep dish, and spread the inside all over with grated bread; put in the mixture, and bake it for three-quarters of an hour.

WAFERS.

Sift half a pound of flour into a pan. Make a hole in the middle, and put in three beaten eggs, a tablespoonful of brandy, a tablespoonful of powdered sugar, a tablespoonful of lard, and a very little salt, not more than will lie on a ten cent piece. Mix all together, adding gradually a little milk, till you have a batter about the thickness of good cream. Then stir in a tablespoonful of rosewater. Let there be no lumps in the batter. Heat your wafer iron on both sides, in a clear fire, but do not allow it to get red hot. Then grease the inside with a brush dipped in lard, or a clean rag with some butter tied up in it. Then put in the batter, allowing about two tablespoonsful to each wafer. Close the iron, and in baking turn it first on one side and then on the other. When done, sprinkle the wafers with powdered sugar, and roll each one up, pressing the edges together while warm, so as to make them unite. A little practice will soon show you the proper degree of heat, and the time necessary for baking the wafers. They should be but slightly colored, and of an even tint all over.

BREAD FRITTERS.

Boil a quart of milk with cinnamon and sugar to your taste. When done, stir in a tablespoonful of rosewater. Cut some slices of bread into a circular shape. Soak them in milk till they have absorbed it; then drain them. Have ready some yolks of eggs well beaten. Dip the slices of bread into it, and fry them in butter. Serve them up stewed with powdered sugar.

CROQUETTES.

Take a pound of powdered sugar, a pound of butter, half a pound of wheat flour, and half a pound of Indian meal; mix all together, and add the juice and grated peel of a large lemon, with spice to your taste. Make it into a lump of paste; then put it into a mortar, and beat it hard on all sides; roll it out thin and cut it into cakes with the edge of a tumbler, or with a tin cutter; flour a shallow tin pan; lay the cakes into it, but not close together; bake them about ten minutes; grate sugar over them when done.

MARGUERITES.

Beat together till very light, a pound of butter, and a pound of powdered sugar; sift a pound of flour into a pan; take the yolks only of twelve eggs, and beat them till very thick and smooth. Pour them into the flour, and add the beaten butter and sugar; stir in a grated nutmeg, and a wine-glass of rosewater; mix the whole together, till it becomes a lump of dough; flour your paste board, and lay the dough upon it; sprinkle it with flour; roll it out about half an inch thick, and cut it into round cakes with the edge of a cup; flour a shallow pan, put in the cakes (so as not to touch), and bake them about five minutes in a quick oven. If the oven is too cool, they will run. When the cakes are cool, lay on each a large lump of currant jelly; take the whites of the eggs, and beat them till they stand alone, then add to them by degrees, sufficient powdered sugar to make the consistence of icing, and ten drops of strong essence of lemon. Heap on each cake, with a spoon, a pile of the icing over the currant jelly; set them in a cool oven till the icing becomes firm and of a pale brownish tint. These cakes are very fine.

RISSOLES.

Make some fine paste, and cut it out with the edge of a tumbler. Have ready some minced veal, seasoned in the best manner, or some chopped oysters, or any sort of force meat, and lay some of it on one half of each piece of paste; then turn over it the other half, so as to enclose the meat. Crimp the edges; put some butter into a frying-pan; lay the rissoles into it, and fry them of a light brown. They should be in the shape of a half moon.

TEA CUSTARDS.

Boil a quart of cream or rich milk, and pour it while boiling on three ounces of the best green tea; add two ounces of loaf sugar; cover it and set it away; take eight eggs, and beat them well, leaving out the whites of four; and when the tea is cold, stir in the eggs. Then strain the whole mixture; put it into cups, and bake them in an oven with water. Grate sugar over the top of each.

POTATOE FLOUR.

Potatoe flour is excellent for sponge cake, and other things which require extraordinary lightness. It is also good for young children and for convalescent sick persons. Take the best and most mealy potatoes; pare them, and wash them through several waters. Then rasp or grate them over a tureen half full of cold water. Continue to grate the potatoes till the lower half of the tureen is filled with the pulp, so that the water may rise to the top. The mealy part of the potatoes will sink to the bottom, while the remainder or the useless part will rise to the surface. When nothing more rises, pour off the water carefully, and dry the flour which you find at the bottom. When quite dry, pound it in a mortar to a fine powder, and sift it through a sieve. Potatoe flour is much lighter than that of wheat.

CHEESE OMELET.

Grate some rich cheese, and mix it gradually with your eggs while beating them; season with salt and pepper; melt some butter in a frying-pan; put in your omelet, and fry it first on one side, and then on the other. When you dish it up, fold it over in half.

STEWED CUCUMBERS.

Lay your cucumbers in cold water for half an hour; then pare them, and cut them into slips about as long as your little finger; take out the seeds; then boil the cucumbers a few minutes, with a little salt. Take them out and drain them well. Put into a stew-pan some butter rolled in flour, and a little cream; stew your cucumbers in it for ten minutes; when you take them off, stir in the yolks of two beaten eggs; and if you choose, a teaspoonful of vinegar.

LOBSTER PIE.

Having boiled your lobster, take out the meat from the shell, season it with salt, mustard, cayenne pepper, and vinegar, and beat it well in a mortar. Then stir in a quarter of a pound of butter, the yolks of two beaten eggs, and two ounces or more of grated bread crumbs. Make some puff-paste, put in the mixture, and cover it with a lid of paste ornamented with leaves or flowers of the same. Bake it slowly.

TURKEY PUDDINGS.

Mince thirty small onions and mix them with an equal quantity of bread crumbs that have been soaked in milk. Chop an equal quantity of the flesh of cold turkey; mix all together, and pound it very well in a mortar. Pass it through a colander, and then return it to the mortar and beat it again, adding gradually the yolks of six hard eggs, and a pint of cream or half a pound of butter; season it to your taste with salt, mace and nutmeg. Have ready some skins, nicely cleaned as for sausages; fill the skins with the mixture, and tie up the ends. Then simmer your puddings, but do not let them boil. Take them out, drain them, and put them away to get cold. When you wish to cook them for immediate use prick them with a fork, wrap them in buttered paper, and broil them on a gridiron.

FRICASSEE OF FOWLS.

Skin and cut up your fowls, and soak them two

hours in cold water, to make them white. Drain them. Put into a stewpan a large piece of butter, and a tablespoonful of flour. Stir them together till the butter has melted. Add salt, pepper, a grated nutmeg, and a bunch of sweet-herbs. Pour in half a pint of cream, put in the fowls and let them stew three quarters of an hour. Before you send them to the table, stir in the yolks of three beaten eggs, and the juice of half a lemon. To keep the fricassee white, cover it (while stewing) with a sheet of buttered paper laid over the fowls. The lid of the stew-pan must be kept on tightly.

A FINE HASH.

Take any cold game or poultry that you have (you may mix several kinds together); some sausages of the best sort will be an improvement. Chop all together and mix with it bread crumbs, chopped onions and parsley, and the yolks of two or three hard-boiled eggs; put it into a saucepan with a proportionate piece of butter rolled in flour, moisten it with broth, gravy, or warm water, and let it stew gently for half an hour. Cold veal or fresh pork may be hashed in the same manner.

A LEG OF MUTTON WITH OYSTERS.

Rub a leg of mutton all over with salt, and put it on the spit to roast with a clear fire, basting it with its own gravy. When it is nearly done, take it up and with a sharp knife make incisions all over it, and stuff an oyster into every hole. Then put it again before the fire to finish roasting. Before you serve it up, skim the gravy well, and give it a boil with a glass of red wine.

BREAD SAUCE.

Take four ounces of grated stale bread, pour over it sufficient milk to cover it, and let it soak about three quarters of an hour, or till it becomes incorporated with the milk. Then add a dozen grains of black pepper, a little salt, and a piece of butter of the size of a walnut. Pour on a little more milk, and give it a boil. Serve it up in a sauce-boat, and eat it with roast wild fowl, or roast pig.

PEA SOUP.

Take two quarts of dried split peas the evening before you intend making the soup, put them in to lukewarm water, and let them soak all night. In the morning, put the peas into a pan or pot with three quarts of cold water, a pound of bacon, and a pound of the lean of fresh beef. Cut up two carrots, two onions, and two heads of celery, and put them into the soup, with a bunch of sweet herb, and three or four cloves. Boil it slowly five or six hours, till the peas can no longer be distinguished, having lost all shape and form; then strain it and serve it up.

GREEN PEA SOUP.

Make a good beef soup with the proportion of four pounds of lean beef to a gallon of water. Boil it slowly, and skim it well. In another pot boil two quarts of green peas with a little salt, and three or four lumps of loaf sugar. When they are quite soft take them out, strain them from the water, and mash them in a colander till all the pulp drips through. Then stir it into the soup after you have taken it up and strained it. Prepare some toasted bread cut into small squares, lay it in a tureen and pour the soup over it. When you toast bread for soups, stews, &c., always cut off the crust.

OYSTER SOUP.

Take two quarts of oysters; drain them; have ready a dozen eggs boiled hard; cut them in pieces, and pound them in a mortar alternately with the oysters. Boil the liquor of the oysters with a head of celery cut small, two grated nutmegs, a teaspoonful of mace, and a teaspoonful of cloves, with two teaspoonsful of salt, and a teaspoonful of whole pepper. When the liquor has boiled, stir in the pounded eggs and oysters, a little at a time. Give it one more boil, and then serve it up. Salt oysters will not do for soup.

BEEF SOUP.

The best soup is made of the lean of fine fresh beef. The proportion is four pounds of meat to a gallon of water. It should boil at least six hours. Mutton soup may be made in the same manner. Put the meat into cold water, with a little salt; set it over a good fire; let it boil slowly but constantly, and skim it well. When no more fat rises to the top, put in what quantity you please of carrots, turnips, leeks, celery, and parsley, all cut into small pieces; add a few cloves. Grate a large red carrot, and strew it over the top; then continue to let it boil, gently but steadily, till dinner time. Next to the quantity and quality of the meat, nothing is more necessary to the excellence of soup than to keep the fire moderate, and to see that it is boiling all the time, but not too fast. Have ready in the tureen some toasted bread, cut into small squares; pour the soup over the bread, passing it through a sieve, so as to strain it thoroughly. Some, however, prefer serving it up with all the vegetables in it. The soup will be improved by boiling in it the remains of a piece of cold roast beef. Soups made of veal, chickens, &c., are only fit for invalids.

MELTED BUTTER.

Put into a saucepan a quarter of a pound of butter. When quite melted over the fire, throw in a large spoonful of flour, and add a half pint of boiling water, and salt to your taste. Boil it a few minutes, and then put in a teaspoonful of cold water. If intended as sauce for a pudding, stir in at least a glass of white wine, and half a grated nutmeg.

A

COLLECTION OF RECEIPTS

FOR DOMESTIC PURPOSES,

AND VARIOUS OTHER MATTERS, VERY USEFUL.

WITH AN INDEX.

RECEIPTS FOR DOMESTIC PURPOSES.

METHOD OF REARING TURKEYS.

The following curious method of rearing turkeys to advantage is translated from a Swedish book, entitled, Rural Economy:—

"Many of our housewives," says this ingenious author, "have long despaired of success in rearing turkeys, and complain that the profit rarely indemnifies them for their trouble and loss of time, whereas," continues he, "little more is to be done than to plunge the chick into a vessel of cold water the very hour, if possible, but at least the very day that it is hatched, forcing it to swallow at least one whole peppercorn; after which let it be returned to its mother. From that time it will become hardy, and fear the cold no more than a hen's chicken. But it must be remembered that this useful species of fowls are also subject to one particular disorder when they are young, which often carries them off in a few days; when they begin to droop, examine carefully the feathers on the rump, and you will find two or three whose quill parts are filled with blood; upon drawing them the chick recovers, and after that requires no other care than what is commonly bestowed upon poultry that range the court-yard." The truth of these assertions is too well known to be denied; and as convincing proof of the success, it will be sufficient to mention, that three parishes in Sweden have, for many years, followed this method, and gained several hundred pounds by rearing and selling turkeys.

ANOTHER METHOD OF REARING AND FEEDING TURKEYS.—The principal remedy necessary, in the first instance, appears to be a stimulant, to counteract the extreme feebleness which attends young turkeys, more than other fowls, in the earliest stages of their existence; hence a grain of pepper, &c., is usually administered as soon as hatched. But instinct, their infallible guide, it appears, has more successfully directed them to the wild onion, which is proved to be a powerful restorative to their natures, and, in fact, a grand panacea to the race; when they are permitted to ramble, you will see them busily cropping the green blades of the onion with much apparent enjoyment. Small hommony made wet, with the addition of a portion of the wild onion chopped fine, or any other onion tops that can be procured, affords the best and most wholesome food they can have, for several weeks at least, or so long as they are confined to small enclosures. Last spring I witnessed with astonishment the wonderful efficacy of this article of food on a large flock of turkeys, which had been daily and rapidly diminishing during the long rainy season in May. The mortality ceased the first day after their change of food, to the above mixture of hommony and onions; and in two or three days their rapid growth and improvement were visible to every eye. Turkeys are very fond of green food of any kind, particularly lettuce and cabbage. Lettuce and cabbage leaves may be chopped fine, and given them twice a day with good effect, morning and evening. Continue also to feed them on hommony, so long as they may require your care, and I venture to say that the good housewife, without uncommon accidents, will have no reason to complain of the want of a good dish while turkeys are in season.—*Farmer's Reg.*

ANOTHER.—Chickens we all know how to raise; but few of us can rear "a good chance of turkeys." I will tell what I know. Next to chickens, of all poultry they are the easiest raised. When the eggs hatch out let the hens and chickens be confined in a garden, or any other place where the young ones can sun themselves. Let them be fed with hommony for two or three days; then carry them to a rail pen, in a rye, oats, or buckwheat patch; confine the hen, and feed at least three times a day with hommony or small grain. The young ones will soon run about catching insects, and will come to the hen's call. The hen should be thus confined until the turkeys are about half grown; they will range about, but never out of the sound of the mother's call. By this plan we do away with the necessity of having a turkey minder. The young ones are not so liable to injury from hawks or vermin, as when they follow the hen, in her rambles over the plantation; nor are they compelled, in keeping up with the hen, to fatigue themselves more than is good for health.

Great care must be taken to keep the pen dry; the foundation should be made higher, with dry sand, so as to admit of no standing water, and the top should be well covered to keep out the rain.

EGGS AND POULTRY.

Every family, or nearly every family, can, with very little trouble, have eggs in plenty during the whole year; and of all the animals domesticated for the use of man, the common dunghill fowl is capable of yielding the greatest possible profit to the owner

In the month of November, I put apart eleven hens and a rooster, giving them a small chamber in the wood-house, defended from storms, and with an opening to the south. Their food, water, and lime, were placed on shelves convenient for them, with warm nests, and plenty of chalk nest eggs. These hens continued to lay eggs through the winter. From these eleven hens I received an average of six eggs daily during the winter, and whenever any of them was disposed to sit, viz., as soon as she began to cluck, she was separated from the others by a grated partition, and her apartment darkened. These cluckers were well attended, and well fed; they could see, and partially associate through their grates with the other fowls, and as soon as any one of these prisoners began to sing, she was liberated, and would very soon lay eggs. It is a pleasant recreation to feed and tend a bevy of laying hens; they may be tamed so as to follow the children, and will lay in a box. Egg shells contain lime, and in winter, when the earth is bound with frost or covered with snow, if lime is not provided for them, they will not lay; or, if they do, the eggs must of necessity be without shells. Old rubbish lime, from old chimneys and old buildings, is proper, and only needs to be broken for them. They will often attempt to swallow pieces of lime plaster as large as walnuts. I have often heard it said that wheat is the best grain for them, but I doubt it; they will sing over Indian corn with more animation than over any other grain. The singing hen will certainly lay eggs, if she finds all things agreeable to her; but the hen is much of a prude, as watchful as a weasel, and as fastidious as a hypocrite: she must, she will have secresy and mystery about her nest;

all eyes but her own must be averted; follow her, or watch her, and she will forsake her nest, and stop laying. She is best pleased with a box, covered at top, with a back side aperture for light, and a side door by which she can escape unseen.

A dozen dunghill fowls shut up, away from the means of obtaining food, will require something more than a quart of Indian corn a day. I think fifteen bushels a year a fair provision for them; but, more or less, let them always have enough by them; and after they have become habituated to find enough at all times, a plenty in their little manger, they take but a few kernels at a time, except just before retiring to roost, when they will take nearly a spoonful into their crops; but just as sure as their provision comes to them scanted, or irregularly, so surely they will raven up a whole crop full at a time, and will stop laying.

A single dozen fowls, properly attended, will furnish a family with more than two thousand eggs in a year, and one hundred full grown chickens for fall and winter stores. The expense of feeding the dozen fowls will not amount to eighteen bushels of Indian corn. They may be kept in cities as well as in the country, and will do as well shut up the year round as to run at large; and a grated room, well lighted, ten feet by five, partitioned from any stable, or other out-house, is sufficient for the dozen fowls, with their roosting places, nests, and feeding troughs.

At the proper season, viz., in the spring of the year, five or six hens will hatch at the same time, and fifty or sixty chickens should be given to one hen. Two hens will take care of one hundred chickens well enough, until they begin to climb their little stick roosts. They should then be separated from the hens entirely. They will wander less, and do better away from the fowls. I have often kept chickens in my garden; they keep the May bugs and other insects away from the vines.

In cases of confining fowls in summer, it would be well that a room with a ground floor should be chosen. And in a southern climate, the situation for the house should be chosen, so that there might be a good yard enclosed, for the fowls to run at large through the day, and attention should be paid to cleaning the yard and house daily, and the house should be very airy.

HENS' EGGS.

A writer in the Farmer's Cabinet, corroborates a fact mentioned by a writer more than two thousand years ago, viz., that hens' eggs which are nearly round, invariably produce female chickens, and those which are long or pointed produce males.

TO FATTEN FOWLS OR CHICKENS IN FOUR OR FIVE DAYS.

Set rice over the fire, with skimmed milk, only as much as will serve one day. Let it boil till the rice is quite swelled out. Feed them three times a day in common pans, giving them only as much as will quite fill them at once. When you boil fresh, let the pans be set in water, that no sourness may be conveyed to the fowls, as that prevents them from fattening. Give them clean water to drink. By this method the flesh will have a clear whiteness which no other food gives; and when it is considered how far a pound of rice will go, and how much time is saved by this mode, it will be found to be cheap.

New England Farmer.

TO CURE THE GAPES IN CHICKENS.

My little son last spring undertook the management of the poultry, and was much troubled by his young chickens dying off with the above disease. He finally discovered the cause by dissecting one. Numerous long worms about the thickness of a common pin were found in its windpipe. He then took a feather, and stripped it except a small tuft on the end, dipped it into spirits of turpentine, and inserted it into the windpipe of the affected chickens, turning it around two or three times before withdrawing it. It was attended with the most complete success, and appeared to give almost immediate relief. In a few cases it required a repetition. The disease was very soon eradicated from his flock, and he afterward raised more than one hundred and forty chickens. The entrance to the windpipe is on the top of the tongue, and near its root, and may be easily discovered by holding the chicken's bill open a short time.

ANOTHER.—On the subject of the disease of chickens called the gapes, a writer remarks : "On the dissection of chickens dying of this disease, it will be found that the windpipe contains numerous small worms about half an inch in length, and the size of a small cambric needle. On the first glance they would likely be mistaken for bloodvessels. These worms may be dislodged, and the disease cured, by the introduction of tobacco smoke into the mouth until the chicken becomes insensible. In this state it will remain for one or two minutes. The operation may be repeated at pleasure, without endangering life. The first application will usually produce the death or expulsion of the worms, and the removal of the affection ; the second, always."

ANOTHER.—Major Chandler, of Davidson, who is one of the most successful chicken growers of all the country, and who is a gentleman of very superior acquirements on most subjects, says the gapes can be prevented in young chickens by the following simple precaution :—Keep iron standing in vinegar, and put a little of the liquid in the food every few days. From the confidence we have in the Major's experience, we are free to recommend the remedy.

TO PREVENT DOGS FROM SUCKING EGGS.

Take of tartar emetic from four to eight grains, according to the age and strength of your dog ; break the end of an egg, put in the tartar and mix it. If your dog is disposed to suck eggs, he will readily eat it. Confine him from cold water. The next day repeat the dose, which continue to do on each succeeding day until he refuses it, which will probably be the third or fourth day. After this I have never known them guilty of the like offence. Instead of being the destroyer of our good wives' poultry, the same dog becomes their faithful protector.

TO MAKE CAPONS.

To the Editor of the Farmer's Pegister.

HANOVER, August 4, 1838.

Sir,—Your last number has just arrived, and I see in it a communication from some one who signs himself "Rusticus," in regard to capons. He says that he has never seen one in this country, and that every person of his acquaintance who has attempted to make them has failed. Now there are living near me some young men who raise great quantities of fowls, and who for their amusement have performed the operation on several young roosters, and have succeeded in every instance but one, and that failure was owing to the fowl being too large. The capons are much larger than the common roosters. Their plumage I think much richer. They take no notice whatever of the hens, are very cowardly, and have a cluck similar to that of a sitting hen. These gentlemen let me know about a year ago the hour on which they would make some of them. I went down, and found the operation a very simple one, and was able to do it myself after having seen some two or three operations performed. After the next communication of "Civis," if his method does not agree with mine, I will let you have my mode, or method.—S. R. M.

METHOD ADOPTED FOR THE OPERATION.

Take the rooster (which should be about half-grown or nearly so), lay him on the left side with the legs and wings extended; let your assistant hold him in that position; then, after picking away some of the feathers from the right side, with a sharp pen knife, make an incision parallel with the ribs, just below them, about an inch and a half in length, taking care not to injure the intestines; then insert the thumb and fore-finger, and you will feel the testicles attached to the back bone, not more than an inch from the incision, which you can remove with the thumb and finger with care; then sew up the incision in three or four stiches, and rub the wound with a little tar or grease. The fowls should be kept for a few days in a coop, and fed sparingly, after which they can be turned loose.

PLAN FOR AN ICE-HOUSE AND DAIRY.

May 2, 1838.

MR. TUCKER.—For several years past, it has been

my design to erect an ice-house, but I had not found it convenient to do so, until the last fall and winter. I have sought for information as to its construction from all the sources accessible to me, without, however, meeting with exactly what I desired. In Rees's Cyclopædia, the American Farmer, and the Genesee Farmer, are found some directions on that subject, and in page 323 of your last volume, more full directions than I had elsewhere met with, but still defective. Some hints were derived from friends in Kentucky, on all of which I endeavoured to improve, especially in attaching a dairy to the ice-room; and which, from the experience we have had thus far, we consider preferable to a spring-house. The temperature of the dairy being 49°, enables us to keep meats, butter, milk, &c., very cool; and between the two doors leading from the dairy into the ice-room, the temperature being 40°, enables us to keep fresh meats as long as desired, there being several hooks driven into one of these doors on which to hang it. Several shelves are put up in the ends of the dairy, for the convenience of placing such articles as we desire to keep very cool. The space between the two doors leading from the dairy to the ice is about fifteen inches, the temperature of which, as above mentioned, is 40°, and it is only by opening these two doors that access is had to the ice, commencing its use at the bottom, instead of the top, as usual. No straw is used about the ice, the room being filled with ice. The work, to be well done, must be done in the summer or early in the fall. If deferred until the winter, the tan cannot be made dry, or if charcoal be used, it is difficult to have it properly prepared.

A Tennessee Subscriber.

Plan of an Ice-House and Dairy.

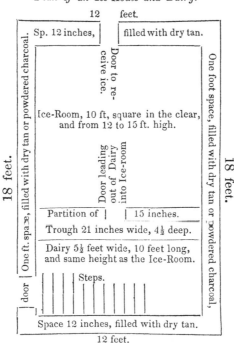

The above is the plan of an ice-house and dairy. The whole length eighteen feet, width twelve feet; the pit sunk six feet in the ground, and to the square above the common surface nine or ten feet. The house to be framed and finished in the common way, and weather-boarded. Another frame is made about two feet less every way, and put up inside of the frame just mentioned, the sills of which rest on the bottom of the pit, ceiled inside, with sleepers in the common way, and the space underneath and between the sleepers filled in with dry tan; floored with two inch plank jointed, and the edges grooved and joints broke, so as to convey the water which drips from the ice into the dairy and into the trough. The partition which separates the dairy from the ice-room is double, and ceiled on both sides the space, which is about twelve to fifteen inches, and is filled with charcoal or dry tan. The ice-room and dairy is intended to be surrounded by dry tan or pulverised charcoal, which, as put in, ought to be rammed. The doors are all double, I mean one inside and one outside, both opening the same way; except the door of entrance into the dairy, the outside one opening to the outside, and the inside opening inside, as usual. The end door to receive the ice is four feet and a half high, and two feet nine inches wide, and the space between the two doors, about a foot, after the ice-room is filled, is packed free of straw. The facings of the doors between the dairy and ice-room are covered with thick woollen selvage, fastened on with small tacks, so as to prevent, as far as possible, the access of warm air. Into one of these doors there are driven several hooks, such as butchers use, on which to hang fresh meat; and the temperature in that open space being 40°, it can be kept there sound and fresh as long as desired. The temperature of the dairy is 49°; the dairy has several shelves, on which to place meats, butter, jars of preserves, &c. &c.; the milk in pans is put in the trough which receives the drippings from the ice. The flight of steps must be narrow, and have a railing as a safeguard. Embankments of clay are made all around the house, to rise perhaps two or three feet above the common surface, so as to carry off the water as it may fall.

The above is a description of one which I have

built, and which answers perfectly. It is better than a spring-house or dairy, and answers the purpose of both. In taking out the ice, we enter the doors leading out of the dairy into the ice-room, beginning, of course, at the bottom of the ice instead of the top, as usual; the ice-room holds about one thousand bushels. The charcoal, when used, ought to be pounded small, or if passed through a bark-mill would perhaps be better; it ought to be fresh. If tan be used it must be dry; and either, as put in, ought to be rammed, and the space between the frames above the ground ought to be from two to four feet, instead of one foot, as mine was made. Care must be taken in constructing the frame, especially the inside one, to give it sufficient height to allow the door of entrance into the dairy to be about six feet. Mine was made too low, and requires those who enter to stoop, and besides causes the dairy to be dark.

The dairy is without a floor. The floor of the ice-room must be somewhat lower where it enters the dairy than at the other end, and the plank forming the floor of the ice-room must project into the dairy over the sleeper a few inches, so that the water running from the floor may fall into the trough, which is made water tight. No straw is used about the ice; the ice-room being filled full. The ice-room is floored above, and covered with charcoal and tan to the thickness of two to four feet.

A PORTABLE ICE-HOUSE.

Take an iron-bound butt or puncheon, and knock out the head, cutting a very small hole in the bottom, about the size of a wine cork; place inside of it a wooden tub, shaped like a churn, resting it upon two pieces of wood, which are to raise it from touching the bottom. Fill the space round the inner tub with pounded charcoal, and fit to the tub a cover, with a convenient handle, having inside one or two small hooks, on which are to be hung the bottles during the operation; place on the lid a bag of charcoal, about two feet square; if the charcoal in this bag is pounded it will answer better; and over all place another cover, which must cover the head of the outer cask. When the apparatus is thus prepared, let it be placed in a cold cellar, and buried in the earth about four-fifths of its length; but though cold, the cellar must be dry; wet ground will not answer, and a sandy soil is the best. Fill the inner tub, or nearly so, with pounded ice; or if prepared in the winter, with snow well pressed down, and the apparatus will be complete. Whenever it is wished to make ice, take off the upper cover, then the sack or bag of pounded charcoal, and suspend the vessel containing the water or liquid to be frozen to the hooks inside of the inner cover; then close up the whole, as before, for half an hour, provided proper care be taken to exclude the external air.

PLAN OF A KENTUCKY BEE-HOUSE.

PLEASANT HILL, November, 30, 1838.

MR. J. BUEL:

SIR,—As I have sufficient room in this letter, I will give you a description of my father's bee-house, which I think preferable to any I have seen, on account of its cheapness and convenience. The building is twelve feet long, eight wide, and seven feet high from the floor to the plate or ceiling (the floor being eighteen inches from the ground), and consists of four posts, which is weather-boarded round, and covered in, so as to prevent the bees from getting in the house; they being confined in six boxes, three on either side of the house, placed fifteen inches one above another. This drawing (fig. 24) represents one side of the house, viewed from the outside.

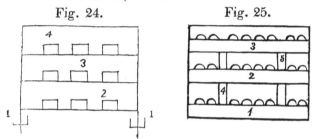

Fig. 24.   Fig. 25.

Fig. 24. No. 1, 1, are copper troughs running round the post, half way between the floor and ground, which are kept filled with water to prevent ants or other insects from getting in the house. No. 2, 3, and 4, are tubes eight inches wide, and one quarter of an inch deep, to convey the bees through the wall into the long boxes, and entering them at the bottom, there being three to each long box. The drawing, fig. 25, represents one side of the house, viewed from the inside. No. 1, 2, and 3, are long boxes, eighteen inches wide, and twelve deep, extending the whole length of the house, with eight holes, four inches square, in each box, upon which is set two gallon caps, with two half inch holes in each, one near the top, the other about the centre of the cap, in which the smoke of a burning rag is blown to drive the bees from the cap into the long box, which can be known by striking the caps when they are all in the long box; a knife or wire should be drawn under the cap, to separate the comb from the box, when the cap of honey may be removed, and an empty one put in its place. Nos. 4 and 5, are tubes, three inches square, to convey the bees from one box to another, that one swarm may do the whole; or if one or more swarms be put in each box, that they may become as one, as they will not have more than one queen when put together, by which they are prevented from destroying themselves by fighting. A house of this description, when the long boxes are filled, will afford, at a moderate calculation, ninety-six gallons of honey in the comb annually.

F. S. FISHER.

ANOTHER.—We have seen a bee-house, the method of constructing which was introduced into our country by Mr. Eber Wilcox, of Salem, and which is said to be a very valuable improvement. Several individuals have tried it with entire success. It consists of a house of brick or wood (of wood standing on blocks, or it might be made with good solid posts set in the ground), say of the size of a common smoke-house, with a door to admit of the entrance of a man. The inside is merely furnished with shelves like an ordinary pantry. The bees pass in and out through several apertures resembling spouts, arranged in rows on each side. These spouts project six inches, and the hole is perhaps two or three inches wide, by from one-eighth to one-half an inch in height. The benefits of this method are said to be these :—The bees never swarm, but continue filling up the house. The honey may be easily taken out when the bees retire to the bottom of the combs in cold weather, and it is said to be an infallible preventive to the worms and the light fingers of the night gentry.—*Courtland Advertiser.*

TAKING HIVES WITHOUT DESTROYING THE BEES.

Having always thought that there was inhumanity in the old plan of destroying the bees in order to take the honey, we determined to try the more humane plan practised by the French of robbing them of their sweets without depriving them of life, and we have put the plan twice into operation the present season with entire success. The method, which is easy, is as follows :—In the dusk of the evening, when the bees are quietly lodged, place a tub near the hive ; then throw the hive over with its bottom upward into the tub ; cover the hive with a clean one, which must be previously prepared by washing its inside with salt and water, and rubbing it with hickory leaves, thyme, or some other aromatic leaves or herbs. Having carefully adjusted the mouth of each hive to the other, so that no aperture remains between them, take a small stick and gently beat around the sides of the full hive for about fifteen minutes, in which time the bees will leave their cells in the lower hive, and ascend and adhere to the upper one. Then gently lift the new hive, with all its little tenants, and place it on the stand from which the other hive was taken. This should be done about midsummer, so as to allow the bees time to provide a new stock of honey for winter's use.

HUNTING BEES.

The manner of hunting bees, as practised in the new settlements, may be familiar to many of the readers of the Genesee Farmer, but perhaps not to all. As advantage is taken of a peculiar instinct, it would, I think, be interesting to those unacquainted with it, to be informed of the process. A tin box is provided, capable of containing about a pint. Into this is put a piece of dry honey-comb; a bottle of honey and water mixed, about half and half, is also provided. The honey is diluted, in order that it may be more readily poured into the dry comb, that the bees may not be so liable to get it upon their wings and will be able to fill themselves more expeditiously. Apparatus for making a fire may also be necessary. With these the hunter proceeds to a newly cleared field, at a distance from any hive of domestic bees; and having poured a little of the composition into the comb, he proceeds to search among the wild flowers for a bee. If one can be found, he is caught in the box by shutting the lid over him. As soon as he becomes still, the lid is carefully removed, when he will be found busily filling himself with honey. When he rises he must be watched in order to ascertain his course. After making one or two circuits about the box, he will fly off in a straight course to his home. After an absence of a few minutes, say five or ten, he will return, bringing with him two or three of his companions. These will soon fill themselves, go home, and return again with a number more. Thus they will continue to increase in number till, in the course of half an hour, there will be one hundred or more in the box. By that time the line will be ascertained with precision. The lid is now shut over as many as possible, and the box is removed on the line to the edge of the woods, where it is again opened. The line will soon be found at the new station, as before, and thus the box is removed from station to station until the whole tree is either discovered or passed. If the tree be passed the line of course will be retrograde. A small pocket spyglass is a convenient thing for searching the tops of trees, as it requires a good eye to see a bee at that distance. If a bee cannot be found to commence operations with, a little honey is burned on a stone; and if a wandering bee happens to be near, he will be attracted by the smell. The proper time for hunting bees is on a fair warm day in the month of September or October. During the summer months, when food for bees is to be found everywhere, they will not traverse. If a bee-tree is in the neighbourhood of a sugar camp, bees will be found about the tree in the time of making sugar. They will traverse well in the spring.—*Genesee Farmer.*

FISH PONDS.

MR. HOLMES.—Perhaps it is not generally known that many kinds of fish at present found in salt water may be taken thence to fresh water, and that they will not deteriorate in flavour. They may thus be transplanted into our fresh-water ponds, where they will speedily multiply, and become not only gratifying to the palate, but actually a source of profit. Experiments have been made in Europe and in this country, and the fact is there rendered beyond dispute, that flounders, bass, cod, mackerel, and eels (and to this list may be added crabs, oysters, muscles and shrimps), all live and do well in fresh water. Many of them, when thus transferred, improve in size and delicacy. The expense of supplying a pond with them is a mere trifle; and what lover of fresh fish will not be willing to cast in his mite to effect the stocking of any pond near him with such inhabitants?

BUTTER MAKING, AS PRACTISED BY S. M. WEEKS, OF VT.

The butter is salted and worked when it comes

from the churn; worked again the next day without cold water in any of the processes, and then packed tight in tubs lined with bags, previously saturated with beeswax, and covered on the top with clean pickle. The great requisites in preserving and making good butter are; 1st. That everything should be cleanly in the whole process. 2nd. That milk should be kept at a proper temperature, say from 45° to 55°, while the cream is separating. 3rd. That the cream should be taken off and churned before its quality is impaired. 4th. That its temperature should be from 55° to 65° when put into the churn, and the churning should be moderate and uniform. 5th. That salt, of the best quality (say alum salt made fine), in sufficient quantity to suit the palate, should be blended with it in the first working, and the butter-milk completely got out by the butter-ladle. 6th. That the working of the butter should be repeated at the end of twenty-four hours, when the salt has become completely dissolved, and all the liquid extracted. 7th. That it should be packed without more salt to make it weigh, in stone jars, in wooden firkins or tubs, such as will not impart to it any taint or bad flavour, and in such a manner as will totally exclude the atmosphere. Butter made in this way will be of fine flavour; and if put down and kept in this way, the flavour will be preserved to an almost indefinate period, if kept in a temperature below 70°; water mixed either with the milk, the cream, or the butter, and especially soft water, adds nothing to, but materially abstracts from richness of flavour. We have no doubt of the position of Mr. Weeks being correct, that milk, skimmed at three several times, will give three qualities of butter; that taken off first being the rcihest and most valuable.

NOTE.—When there is a difficulty of obtaining good butter quick in churning, it is said, by adding a tablespoonful of good vinegar to four gallons of cream it may be obtained in a few minutes.

PATENT BUTTER.

A Prussian nobleman, of high rank, and the possessor of a large landed estate, has received from the Emperor letters patent, as a reward for discovering a new method of making butter, which may be of importance to dairy-women in this country. The process consists in boiling, or rather simmering the milk, for the space of fifteen minutes, in its sweet state, taking care not to burn it; and then churning it in the usual manner. It is said no difficulty ever occurs in making butter immediately, and of a quality far superior to that made from milk which has undergone vinous fermentation. Butter made in this manner is also said to preserve its flavour and sweetness much longer than butter made in the ordinary manner. The milk likewise being left sweet, is considered of nearly the same value as before churning, and far more healthy on account of its having the animalculæ, or whatever else it may have contained, destroyed. The ease with which the experiment may be made, should induce all to give it a fair trial.
Silk Culturist.

STRONG BUTTER.

We wish our dairy-women would learn one thing, viz., to work out all buttermilk from the butter they make, and prepare it in such a manner that it will keep sweet during the year; and we wish our butter merchants would learn two things, viz., how to lay butter down in such a manner that it shall not become strong or rancid, and to discriminate between good butter and poor, and pay a price accordingly. We feel rather sour-croutish on this subject, having had our throats rancified for a long time with what was once butter, till our very disposition begins to grow rather unsavory. We have actually had to swallow one or two anathemas against careless dairy-women, and the indiscriminating buyer and vender of half-churned, half-worked, and ought to be half-priced article, called in common language, through pure courtesy, butter. The art of making good butter is exceedingly simple, and may be reduced to a few rules. In the first place keep every utensil clean and sweet; then be careful to churn the cream before it is too old; churn it well, till the buttermilk is separated from the butter; work out all the buttermilk, and then salt with good Turk's Island or rock salt. We dislike the Liverpool salt: it will not keep the butter pure and sweet; it contains Glauber salts, sulphate of magnesia, muriate of lime, and other impurities.

SALTING BUTTER.

It is not unfrequently that we hear complaints, which, we have no doubt, are well founded, that much of the butter for sale in our market is strongly rancid and unfit for use. But where lies the fault? Our dairy-women are not altogether chargeable with the evil; many of them know their duty and do it faithfully, as far as the manufacture of the article is concerned. When it is first made, it is pure and sweet, and they do all in their power to preserve it in that state; but, in spite of all their efforts, after it has remained a short time it will become strong, bitter, and disagreeable. From our own experience we are induced to believe, that the greatest part of the fault is in the salt which is used in it. We are never able to preserve butter in its purity, for any length of time, salted with the Liverpool salt; while the butter made in the same way, and salted with the ground rock salt, has been kept a year, retaining the same sweet and pleasant flavour it possessed when first taken from the churn. That the fine Liverpool salt is not fit to be used to preserve meat or butter is a fact not so generally known as it should be; its convenience for use, and white texture, induce people to buy it. But if, instead of this, they would purchase the ground rock salt, notwithstanding they would have to pay a higher price, they would be gainers in the end. Dr. Mitchell, of New York, who is one of the best chemists in our country, analyzed the Liverpool salt, and, after thoroughly examining its properties, he condemns the use for any purpose whatever, and says the loss of property consequent upon the employment of this salt is prodigious. Experience, year after year, has proved it to be incapable of preserving our beef from corruption. Often has this important article of food been found to be tainted the very autumn in which it has been packed in barrels; besides the sacrifice of property, we find that the employment of Liverpool salt, in the packing of beef and pork, leaves them liable to corrupt; and the consequences of this corruption are pestilential exhalations, stirring up yellow fever and other malignant distempers in the neighborhoods, cities, and vessels where the bodies of those slaughtered animals are deposited.

The butter of New York market has also been rendered worse, if not absolutely spoiled, by the same kind of salt. Beguiled by its fine and showy exterior, the citizens have used it extensively in our country, famous for grazing and dairies. In many cases it has supplanted the old-fashioned coarse or sun-made salt. Whenever the substitution has been made, it has been with a pernicious effect. The butter so salted does not keep so well, and loses its agreeable scent. The difference between butter put up with this salt, and with natural crystallized salt, is so great, that our wholesale and retail grocers can distinguish it at once by the smell on piercing or opening a firkin. The sweet flavour and nice odour which pure sea salt gives is altogether wanting in that which is seasoned with the other. And thus as Liverpool salt is the remote agent of so much loss, damage, and misery to the United States, it is high time to cease both to buy and consume it. In its stead, salt from the bay of Biscay, Portugal, Isle of May, or the Bahamas, may be employed with perfect safety. The fault of Liverpool salt, and of all other salt obtained from sea water by force of fire or by boiling, is its admixture with foreign ingredients, known by the technical names of slack and bittern. These usually adhere to sea salt in considerable quantities. They have no antiseptic virtues, but possess a directly contrary effect. Sea salt, formed by natural evaporation and crystallization, has very little mixture with these foul and foreign ingredients.—*Maine Farmer*.

PACKING BUTTER.

Take a stone pot, or jar, that will hold thirty or forty pounds; clean it thoroughly, and wash it in cold strong brine; take of new sweet butter, well made and free from buttermilk; work it well, and put a layer of it, a few inches in thickness, in the jar; beat it down solid with a wooden beater, turning off the milk that will escape occasionally; then repeat the process, until the pot is filled within an inch and a half of the top with butter thoroughly pounded down; on the top of this pour one inch of clear brine, made by dissolving salt in warm water, and put on when cold; cork the jar tight, and tie over a cloth or piece of buckskin; keep the jar at a low temperature, and the butter will keep good and sweet for an indefinite length of time, only examining it occasionally to see that it is covered with the brine, and renewing it if necessary.

CURING PORK.

In the New York Farmer, I noticed a receipt for making Knickerbocker pickle, for beef or pork. I will give mine, which I have used for twenty-six years with uniform success, and I will tell how and where I got it. In August, 1805, I lodged from Saturday to Monday, with an innkeeper in Cherry Valley, N. Y., who was also a farmer. On the table for Sunday's dinner there was a fine piece of pickled pork, boiled the day before. I thought it the most delicious I ever ate. I requested my host to give me his receipt for curing it, which is as follows:—As soon as my hogs are dressed, and cool enough to be cut, I pack the side pieces in a cask or barrel, with plenty of salt on all sides of each piece: and when my cask is full, I immediately roll it to the pump, and pump in water until I can see the water cease to sink in the vessel, or to moisten the salt on the top of the cask. I then lay a flat stone, as large as the vessel will receive, on the top, so as to keep the pork always under the pickle; I put it in my cellar, covered so as to exclude the flies and air, and there it remains until a piece is wanted. Care must be taken to keep the meat under the pickle, otherwise it will rust. Here is the whole secret of making good pickled pork for family use.

Note.—Alum or rock salt made fine should be made use of for rubbing and putting down the meat in the cask, and if the pork is bloody it would be well to salt the meat well with fine salt on boards for forty-eight hours to let all the blood drain off, and then pack down as above.

TO CURE BACON—BY A VIRGINIAN—SAID TO BE EQUAL TO THE BURLINGTON METHOD OF CURING HAMS.

First salt the pork by giving it a pretty good salting with fine salt, and pack it away on boards, with a slope sufficient to let the brine run off. In this situation it lies eight or ten days, when it is taken up, and each piece wiped dry with a coarse cloth, and to each ham and shoulder is added a heaping teaspoonful of the best crystallized saltpetre, by sprinkling over them, and rubbing it well in with the hand. It is then salted well again, and packed away in tight casks, as it then may be an advantage to retain or preserve all the brine you can: whereas the first brine I have found from experience to be of great injury, as it tends to putrescence, and should by no means be re-absorbed by the meat lying in it after being extracted by the salt, as I conceive it to be that which so easily produces the bugs and skippers in the meat after it has been smoked. The time of putting on the saltpetre is of much more importance than is supposed by those who have not made the trial; for if put on at the first salting, the meat is always dry, hard, and too salt. On giving the meat a second salting I add to the salt as much brown sugar as will moisten or damp it, and as much of the common red pepper as will give the salt quite a red appearance. The pods are first dried before a fire, or on a griddle, and then pounded fine in a mortar. The meat then lies about five or six weeks, except farther south, where the climate is more moderate; then four weeks will answer, except the meat be very large and the weather continue very cold. It is then taken out, and each piece rubbed well with hickory ashes, and hung up to smoke with the hock downward, which prevents its dripping, and thereby retains its juice. The coarse alum salt, made fine, should be made use of at the second salting, as it is much more effectual in preserving the meat sweet and pure. Should there not be sufficient pickle from the last salting to cover the hams and shoulders, a strong brine may be made with alum salt, enough to answer the purpose, by boiling it well—observing to skim it while boiling as long as any scum arises, and the brine should not be put on till cold. It is not very essential to add the saltpetre to the middlings, or to cover them with pickle, as they are easily preserved without, particularly when the ribs or bones are taken out, which should be the case when they are large, say when the hogs are over one hundred pounds in weight. It may be well to let the meat hang one day to dry before a smoke is made, which should be done with hickory or oak chips raked up from the wood pile; and in order to prevent a blaze or too much heat, it would be well to add or mix a little saw-dust made from the hickory or oak wood, or tanner's bark might do very well to add with the oak chips. After the meat is sufficiently smoaked, which might be in the course of four or five weeks, if regularly attended to, it might be taken down and packed away in casks or boxes, with charcoal made fine, covering the meat entirely with it; and in the course of the summer it might be taken out once or twice, and examined, and sunned if necessary. The hams and shoulders might be preserved in a good state during the summer if they were sewed up in good stout linen bags, painted or lined, provided it was done early in the spring, before any flies made their appearance. Middlings might remain hung up in the smoke house, and keep very well by taking them down two or three times to sun, or by making a smoke occasionally under them on a damp day.

TO CURE HAMS SO AS TO PRESERVE THEM FROM FLIES.

From the Farmers' Cabinet.

For a score of hams, take about three quarts of salt, one pint of molasses, quarter of a pound of black pepper, and two ounces of saltpetre pulverized; mix well together; lay the hams on a table with the rind downwards; rub the mixture over them with the hand, taking care to apply it to every part where there is no rind; let them lay a week, and rub them over with clear salt, which continue once a week for four or five weeks, according to the size of the hams; they are then ready to smoke; or if you choose, after the mixture is sufficiently struck in, put them into brine for two or three weeks before you smoke them; and when smoked, hang them in a dry place. When a ham is cut for use, hang or lay it where you please, the flies will not touch it. We have practised this method for several years, and have no reason to abandon it.

HAMBOROUGH PICKLE.

The following constitutes the famed Hamborough pickle, which has been found to preserve meat effectually, in hot as well as in cold climates:—

Six pounds of alum salt, eight ounces of brown sugar, and six ounces of saltpetre. Dissolve these articles by boiling in four gallons of water. In this pickle, when perfectly cold, keep any kind of meat sunk and stopped closely. The pickle will also keep beef from being hard and too salt when boiled. Tongues, veal, or mutton, for smoking, should not remain in the pickle longer than ten days. Beef, or tongues, when taken out of the pickle for boiling, should be kept twenty-four hours in cold water, and then drained before they are boiled.

TO PRESERVE BEEF TENDER AND SWEET THROUGHOUT THE YEAR.

For one hundred weight of beef, prepare the following: Four quarts of coarse alum salt, made fine; four pounds of brown sugar, and four ounces of saltpetre. Mix these articles well together; then rub your meat with it, and pack closely in the barrel. Sufficient pickle will soon be made in the cask by this process. By no means use any water, as it will spoil the meat when the weather becomes warm. If at any time a scum rise on the barrel, skim it off, and sprinkle into it a little fine salt, which will preserve the pickle.— Some persons, fearing their beef will be injured in warm weather, take out the pickle and boil it. This is wrong, as it will harden the beef, and entirely change its flavour.

TO PRESERVE MEAT FRESH FOR A FEW DAYS.

Put the meat into the water running from a spring.

It will sink. Examine it daily; when it begins to rise from the bottom it must be used. It will be found perfectly sound and tender, and may be boiled or roasted. Meat may be preserved in this manner three or four days in summer-time free from taint.— The outside will appear somewhat whitened, but the flavour is not injured. It would be advisable to have a box or tub with a cover, into and out of which the water shall have free passage, which may be put either inside or outside of the spring-house.

TO RESTORE TAINTED MEAT.

If your meat be tainted, take it out of the pickle; wash it so as to cleanse it of the offensive pickle. Then wash your barrel well, either with a solution of lime or ashes, after which repack it, and between every layer of meat put a layer of charcoal until your barrel be full; then make a fresh pickle strong enough to bear an egg, and fill up your barrel. As you repack your pieces, it would be well to rub each piece with salt. Let it remain a week or ten days, and the taint will have disappeared, and the meat be restored to its original sweetness.

TO SWEETEN MEAT, FISH, ETC., THAT ARE TAINTED.

When meat, fish, &c., from intense heat or long keeping, are likely to pass into a state of corruption, a simple and pure mode of keeping them sound and heathful is, by putting a few pieces of charcoal, each the size of an egg, into the pot wherein the fish or flesh is to be boiled. Among others, an experiment of this kind was tried upon a turbot, which appeared too far gone to be eatable. The cook, as advised, put three or four pieces of charcoal, each the size of an egg, under the strainer, in the fish kettle. After boiling the proper time, the turbot came to the table perfectly sweet and clean.

TO MAKE SOFT SOAP.

Take five bushels of ashes, damp them thoroughly on the ground, and let them stand from five hours to two days, as may be convenient. Then make up the heap in an oblong form, open the middle, and put in three pecks of perfectly fresh lime, and sprinkle about three or four quarts of water over it, and cover up. Observe to use hot water in very cold weather. In large experiments cold water will answer in any weather. In half an hour the lime will heat and burst open the heap of ashes, when the whole must be well and quickly mixed, and put into the ley tub to the depth of one foot, and beaten moderately; another layer of ashes, the same depth as the first, is then to be added and beaten as before, and so on until the tub is filled within six inches of the top; water is then to be poured in steadily until the ashes are nearly or entirely spent. The ley must be of a strength scarcely sufficient to float a newly laid egg: four gallons of this ley are to be put into a large kettle, and thirty or forty pounds of fat or grease added, and well stirred over a gentle heat. When it is perceived that the sharp taste of the mixture is lost, more ley is to be added occasionally, until the soap becomes transparent and very thick, and toward the last of the operation, the liquid must be made to boil briskly. When the soap is made let it stand for a day, when, if it does not grow thin in that time, no apprehensions need be excited as to the occurrence of that circumstance. The kettle should be covered, and should hold more liquid than it is intended to boil, to give room for a brisk ebullition toward the close.

TO MAKE HARD SOAP.

Mild ley is to be used. When the soft soap is finished, and the mixture still tolerably hot, add sea salt (or alum salt), until the ley drops clear from the soap. If it closes, add more salt, and at the same time slacken the fire; then boil until the froth becomes as light as a feather. Draw the fire, and pour in salt and water into the mixture to cool it, observing to make a rapid stream, and not to let any drops fall in turning the bucket. When the soap is too strong of the alkali, it will not grain : in that case, add clean fat by degrees until it granulates, stirring it all the time over a gentle heat : when it boils, no more fat need be added. It is to be observed that if the ashes have been too tightly pressed in the ley tub, the ley will not filtrate ; and if they have not been sufficiently pressed, the water will run foul. In the first case, the ashes may be loosened with a long iron skewer ; in the latter, they must remain some hours to settle, and also be pressed.

TO MAKE COLD SOAP.

The leach tub, or hogshead, must be covered at the bottom with straw and sticks ; then put in a bushel of ashes, then two or three quarts of unslacked lime, upon which you must throw two quarts of boiling water to excite fermentation and slack ; put in another bushel of ashes, and as much more lime and water, and continue to do so until your vessel is full ; put in hot water until you can draw off the ley, after which the heat of the water is not of much consequence. You must have at least two-thirds of a bushel of lime to a hogshead, if you wish your soap to be made quick : one hogshead of ashes will make two barrels of soap. When you draw off your ley, you must keep the first two pailsful by themselves, and the next two in another vessel, and the third two in another vessel still; then weigh twenty-nine pounds of clear strained grease, or of scraps without straining thirty pounds, put into a large kettle with three pounds of resin; then pour over it one pailful of ley from the first drawn vessel, and one from the second drawn vessel, put it over the fire and let it boil twenty minutes: be careful to add no ley over the fire, but swing off the crane if it is in danger of boiling over; put it into your barrel, and put in one pailful of ley from the third drawn vessel, and give it a good stir: then weigh your grease for another barrel, and take the ley remaining in the vessels in the same manner as for the first barrel; then draw off your weak ley, and fill up the vessels as fast as possible, remembering to put half in each barrel, that they may be equally strong: if your leach run through fast, you may have your barrels full in an hour, and so hard that you can hardly stir them. You must stir it after you put in your ley, till your barrel is full. Fourteen quarts of melted grease is the quantity for a barrel.

A SIMPLE METHOD FOR MAKING SOAP.

To thirty-two gallons of ley, of strength just sufficient to bear an egg, add sixteen pounds of clean melted grease, which, by being placed in the hot sun, and occasionally stirred, will, in a few days, produce a soap of the first quality.

MAKING DIPPED CANDLES.

The tallow, when melted, should be ladled into a wooden vessel of convenient width and depth, which has been previously heated by filling it with boiling water for an hour or more. Fill the vessel within an inch of the top with melted tallow, and keep it that height by adding hot tallow or hot water. By this means the candles will be kept of a full size at the top, and not taper off to a point, as is often seen with the country candles. The tallow, when used for dipping candles, should not be too hot. A temperature that will allow the finger to be dipped in without burning, is sufficiently hot, and at this temperature the tallow will take on the wicks very fast. The wicks should be lowered into the melted tallow very gradually, and should be lifted out of the tallow so slowly that when the bottoms of the candles are clear from the surface of the melted tallow, no tallow will run off them. When the candles are raised quick out of the melted tallow, the tallow will run off the candles in a stream; whereas if the candles are raised out slowly, not a particle of tallow will fall from the candles. A few trials will satisfy any person in this matter. If the tallow is boiling hot, the wick will not take on the tallow to any considerable extent. When candles are raised out of the tallow rapidly, the candles will be large at the bottom, and the tallow will extend below the wick, so that when burnt in the candlestick a piece of the candle will have no wick in it; and therefore, for burning, will be useless. Where people have no suitable wooden vessel, an iron vessel will answer for a dipping vessel. When tallow has been thoroughly melted over the fire, should it be dirty or impure, throw into it, while hot, a small quantity of finely powdered alum, and in a short time a scum will be seen rising to the surface, in appearance like dirty froth. Skim this off as it rises. This scum will rise for half an hour or more. These directions are plain and easily complied with, and one trial will be satisfactory. Persons, by following the directions, will save more than one half the usual labour of making candles, besides having better candles. I speak from abundant experience, and therefore with full confidence. E. M.

NOTE.—Prepare your wicks about half the usual size, and wet them thoroughly with spirits of turpentine, put them in the sun until dry, and then mould or dip your candles. Candles thus made, last longer, and give a much clearer light. In fact they are nearly or quite equal to sperm, in clearness of light. We have used candles of this kind, and can therefore recommend them with confidence.

A NEW WAY TO MAKE CANDLES.

We have been shown a candle, about the size of a broom straw, which makes a very brilliant light, and is as durable as the tallow candle. As this is the age for economy in everything, it may not be amiss for us to tell our readers how to make them. Take one pound of beeswax, and a fourth of a pound of soft turpentine from the tree, melt them together, strain them; take your wick of the desired length, and stretch it as you would in making a plough line; then take the composition in a thin waiter, and hold the wick down in it as you apply it from end to end; this done three times will complete the operation. The above proportion of the ingredients is sufficient for a wick forty yards long. *Chambers (Ala.) Herald.*

TO DYE COTTON YARN A DEEP BLUE.

Take one pound of logwood, chipped fine, or pounded; boil it in a sufficient quantity of water until all the substance is out of it; then take about half a gallon of the liquor, and dissolve in it half an ounce of alum, and one ounce of verdigris; boil your yarn in the logwood water one hour, stirring and keeping it loose. Take out your yarn, mix the half gallon that contains the verdigris and alum; then put your yarn into the mixture, and boil it four hours, stirring it and keeping it loose all the time, and taking it out once every hour to give it air; after which dry it, then boil it in soap and water, and it is done. The above will dye six pounds of yarn an elegant deep blue; after which put in as much yarn into the same liquor, and boil it three hours, stirring it as before, and you will have a good pale blue; or boil hickory bark in your liquor, and you will have an elegant green.

TO COLOUR GREEN.

Take half a pound of oil of vitriol, one ounce of indigo, pulverized; put them in a bottle, shake it repeatedly three or four days; then put it in a hickory bark dye, with two pounds of alum. This mixture will cover twelve pounds of yarn; it is to be simmered over the fire several hours, frequently taking it out to air on a pole over the kettle: you can dye it in iron, copper, or brass. When the yarn is dry, wash it in cold water; the hickory dye is to be taken off the fire, when the mixture is put in out of the bottle, or it will run over; for the hickory dye must be boiling hot when it is put in.

TO COLOUR RED.

To three pounds of yarn, take one pound of alum, and one pound of madder; dissolve your alum in a sufficient quantity of water to cover your yarn; scald it well in that water; then rinse it well in pure water;

mix wheat bran and water to the consistence of thin gruel, a sufficient quantity to cover the yarn well; mix the madder well in this preparation; put in the yarn, and boil two or three hours, stirring and keeping it loose in the vessel. If you do not wish it deep, take it out in a very short time; but if you wish a deep colour, let it remain several hours. Rinse it in cold water after letting it air. The bran must be boiled the night before, and a crock, part full, taken out and strained, and then put in to raise the rest; strained in the morning, and that in the crock mixed with the other before put into boil.

TO DYE RED, WITH REDWOOD.

One pound of redwood (chipped fine), two ounces of alum, powdered; the redwood must stand twenty-four hours in river or spring water; then boil it well, and after straining, mix your alum and aquafortis, and boil it well for several hours. Mix one ounce aquafortis, one ounce block tin, in a tumbler, and set it in the sun about one hour. The above will colour two pounds of yarn; after being dried, wash out with soft soap.

TO DYE CRIMSON COLOUR.

To two gallons of the juice of pokeberries, when they are quite ripe, add half a gallon of strong cider vinegar, to dye one pound of wool, which must be first washed very clean with hard soap; the wool, when wrung dry, is to be put into the vinegar and pokeberry juice, and simmered in a copper vessel for one hour; then take out the wool and let it drip a while, and spread it in the sun. The vessel must be free from grease of any kind.

TO DYE PINK.

Two ounces cochineal, two pounds of cream tartar, one pound of alum, the whole put in a kettle of soft water; then put in six pounds of clean yarn, and boil it well; not to be washed after being dried.

TO COLOUR YELLOW.

Take three fourths of hickory bark, with the outside shaved off, and one fourth of black oak bark done in the same manner; boil them well together in a bell-metal kettle until the colour is deep; then add alum sufficient to make it foam when stirred up; then put your yarn in, and let it simmer a little while; take it out and air it two or three times, having a pole over the kettle to hang it on so that it may drain in the kettle; when dry, rinse it in cold water.

COLOURING FLANNEL.

Take black alder bark, boil it well, then skim or strain it well; wet the cloth in a pretty strong ley, and dip it into the alder liquor: let it remain till cool enough to wring, and you will have an indelible orange colour. The better the cloth, the better the colour.

NANKEEN COLOUR.

A pailful of ley, with a piece of copperas half as big as a hen's egg boiled in it, will colour a fine nankeen colour, which will never wash out.

POKEBERRY DYE.

Mr. Moses Lindo, of South Carolina, in 1764, boiled three quarters of a pint of the juice, with a pint of rain water, about a quarter of an hour. He then took pieces of flannel, and numbered them one and two, boiled them in alum in a separate pot, for a quarter of an hour, and rinsed them in cold water. He then dipped the flannel No. 1. into the pot of prepared juice, and after it had simmered five minutes, he rinsed it in cold water; a crimson dye was fixed in the piece superior to the colour of the juice itself. He then dipped the flannel No. 2. in the juice; and washing his hands, which were stained with the juice, in lime water, he found the colour change to a bright yellow. He then threw a wine glass full of lime water into the pot where No. 2. was simmering, which turned both juice and flannel to a bright yellow. Thus he found that alum fixed the crimson, and lime water the yellow colour.

METHOD OF CLEANSING SILK, WOOLLEN, AND COTTON GOODS, WITHOUT DAMAGE TO THE TEXTURE OR COLOUR.

Take raw potatoes in the state they are taken out of the earth, wash them well, then rub them on a grater over a vessel of clean water to a fine pulp, pass the liquid matter through a coarse sieve into another tub of clean water; let the mixture stand till the fine white particles of the potatoes are precipitated, then pour the mucilaginous liquor from the fecula, and preserve this liquor for use. The article to be cleansed should then be laid upon a linen cloth on a table, and having provided a clean sponge, dip it in the potatoe liquor, and apply this sponge thus wet upon the article to be cleansed, and rub it well upon it with repeated portions of the potatoe liquor, till the dirt is perfectly separated, then wash the article in clear water several times to remove the loose dirt; it may afterwards be smoothed or dried. Two middle sized potatoes will be sufficient for a pint of water.

The coarse pulp which does not pass the sieve is of

great use in cleansing worsted curtains, tapestry, carpets, or other coarse goods. It is also useful in cleansing oil paintings, or furniture that is soiled. Dirty painted wainscots may be cleaned by wetting a sponge in the liquor, then dipping it in a little fine clean sand, and afterwards rubbing the wainscot therewith.

TO CLEAN SILK STOCKINGS.

Wash your stockings first in white soap liquor lukewarm, to take out the rough dirt; then rinse them in fair water, and work them well in a fresh soap liquor; make a third soap liquor pretty strong and hot, in which put a little stone blue, wrapped in a flannel bag, till your liquor is blue enough, then wash your stockings well therein, and wring them. Let them be dried so that they may remain a little moist, then stove them with brimstone; after which put upon a wooden leg two stockings, one upon the other, observing that the two fronts, or outsides, are face to face; then polish them with a glass.

TO TAKE MILDEW OUT OF LINEN.

Take soap, and rub it well; then scrape some fine chalk, and rub that also in the linen; lay it on the grass; as it dries wet it a little, and it will come out at twice doing.

TO TAKE STAINS OUT OF SILK.

Mix together in a phial two ounces essence of lemon, one more of oil of turpentine. Grease and other spots in silk, are to be rubbed gently with a fine rag, dipped in the above composition.

TO TAKE SPOTS OUT OF SILK, LINEN.

Of spirits of turpentine twelve drops, and the same quantity of spirits of wine; grind these with an ounce of pipe-makers' clay, and the spots therewith. You are to wet the composition when you do either silk, linen, or woollen with it. Let it remain till dry, then rub it off, and the stains or spots will disappear. True spirits of salt, diluted with water, will remove iron-moulds from linen; and sal-ammoniac, with lime, will take out the stains of wine.

TO TAKE GREASE OUT OF SILK.

If a little powdered magnesia be applied on the wrong side of silk as soon as the spot is discovered, it is a never failing remedy: the dark spots disappear as if by magic.

ANOTHER.—Magnesia, if you have not French chalk, will effectually remove grease spots from silk, on rubbing it in well; and after standing a while, apply a piece of soft brown paper to the wrong side, on which press a warm iron gently, and what grease is not absorbed by the paper, can be removed by washing the spot carefully with cold water.

TO WASH SILK.

Lay the piece of silk upon a clean board; soap a piece of flannel well, without making it very wet, and with this rub the silk carefully and evenly one way. After having thus cleansed one side of the silk, take a wet sponge and wash the soap; proceed in the same manner to clean the other side, and then wipe the water off each with a clean dry cloth; after which hang it as singly as possible upon a linen horse, and let it dry gradually; when very nearly dry, iron it with a cool box. In this manner we last summer washed a slate-colored dress, which was so dirty with the constant wear of a winter that we did not like to use it even for linings, without endeavoring to remove some of the spots, and we were quite hopeless of its being fit for anything except linings, even when washed; but its brightness was completely restored, and its texture softer than when new.

TO MAKE CALICOES WASH WELL.

Infuse three gills of salt in four quarts of boiling water, and put the calicoes in while hot, and leave them till cold; in this way the colours are rendered permanent, and will not fade by subsequent washing. So says a lady who has frequently made the experiment herself.

TO REMOVE IRON MOULDS FROM LINEN.

Hold the iron mould on the cover of a tankard of boiling water, and rub on the spots a little juice of sorrel and salt; when the cloth has thoroughly imbibed the juice, wash it in ley.

TO REMOVE STAINS BY FRUIT.

These are readily removed from clothes by wetting them, and placing them near lighted brimstone. A few matches will answer the purpose.

TO REMOVE INK SPOTS.

As soon as the accident happens, wet the place with the juice of sorrel, or lemon, or with vinegar, and the best hard white soap.

TO TAKE INK, OR WINE OUT OF LINEN OR WOOLLEN.

Take the juice of lemons, and wet the spot with it several times, letting it dry each time, then wash it with soap and vinegar, and the spot will go out.

TO REMOVE INK SPOTS FROM LINEN.

Lemon juice will effectually remove ink from linen or muslin, if applied before the article has been washed. But as persons in the country may not be able at all times to get a lemon, I would advise them to buy a small bottle of vitriol. A few drops of this acid mixed with pure water, and applied to the spots of ink, will entirely remove them. Great caution must be observed, however, not to suffer any part of the linen or other material, to come in contact with the acid before it is sufficiently diluted: otherwise the texture of the fabric will be destroyed.

TO PREVENT MOTHS.

In the month of April, or before flies or insects make their appearance, beat your fur or woollen garments well with a small cane or elastic stick; then wrap them up in linen, observing not to press the fur garments too hard, and put between the folds some camphor in small lumps; then put your articles in this state in boxes well closed. When the garments are wanted for use, take them out, beat them well as before, and expose them twenty-four hours to the air, which will take away the smell of the camphor.

TO BLEACH BEESWAX.

Melt your wax, and while hot throw it into cold water to reduce it into small pieces, or spread it out into very thin leaves, and lay it out in the sun and air for a few days on linen cloths; then melt it over again, and expose it as before, till the sun and dew have bleached it; then, for the last time, melt it in a kettle, and cast it with a ladle on a table covered over with little round hollow moulds in the form of the casks sold by the apothecaries; but first wet your moulds with cold water, that the wax be the easier got out; lastly, lay it out in the air for two or three days and nights, to make it more transparent and drier.

SIMPLE MEANS OF PURIFYING WATER.

It is not generally known, as it ought to be, that pounded alum possesses the property of purifying water. A large tablespoonful of pulverised alum, sprinkled into a hogshead of water (the water sound at the time), will, after the lapse of a few hours, by precipitating to the bottom the impure particles, purify it, so that it will be found to possess nearly all the freshness and clearness of the finest spring water; a pailful, containing four gallons, may be purified with a single teaspoonful.

HOW TO MAKE A MATTRASS, THAT SHALL NOT SINK IN THE MIDDLE, OR BECOME HARD BY THE WEIGHT OF THE BODY.

To produce this effect, make your mattrass twice as long as usual, double it, sew the two ends together, and arrange the stuffing where it joins the same as the rest. It will then have the form of a roller or double towel, which may be rolled for ever, and will always remain double and folded. When you put it on the bed, it will be the same as two mattrasses one over the other. It takes no more tucking or stuffing for this double mattrass than for two single ones. The advantage of this invention is, that every time the bed is made, you may easily roll the mattrass, so that the part which was under the body may be placed at the head or feet, sometimes above and sometimes below, and successively every part of the mattrass made to pass to those places where the compression is greater; you may even, from time to time, turn it inside out like a stocking, and by this means produce other changes. A mattrass made in this manner lasts much longer, and is much easier to sleep on than one made in the usual way.

TO EXPEL RATS AND MICE.

Take one or more (of either) alive, and baste or wet them well with a mixture of about equal quantities of train oil and tar (the tar alone would be rather too stiff), then let them go. The consequence will be that, feeling so unpleasant, they will run through every hole and avenue hunted by their tribe, and baste and daub the whole family, and render them so uncomfortable, that they will become entirely blind by the tar getting into their eyes, and will run at random; and may be trod on, or knocked over with a stick. This experiment may be relied on as perfectly adapted to the purpose.

TO DESTROY RATS.

Take a few fresh corks, rasp them fine, and fry them in the common way with a little butter or fat; place it, while warm, at the places where rats are plenty, and, if possible, where they may eat the dose undisturbed by any noise; leave no water within their reach, and in a few days not a vestige of the creatures is to be seen. The above plan is more safe than poisoning them.

ANOTHER MODE.—Take a small pine stick, and slightly fasten six or eight fish-hooks to it, the points all one way, and put the stick in the rat holes, so that when they run into the hole they will rub against the hooks, which will catch into the skin, and with a little exertion they clear the hooks from the stick, and go off squealing with the hooks fast in the skin; and a few rats, so hooked, will give warning to others, and they will all soon disappear. Try it, and you will not be disappointed.

TO DESTROY BED-BUGS.

During last summer, being much troubled with bed-bugs, I tried the various means I had heard of to expel them, but I found none of them would answer the purpose. After pouring boiling water on them, I watched them, and perceived, though they lay apparently dead for a time, that most of them would revive. The same happened when I applied spirits of turpentine, corrosive sublimate, &c. My patience was at last exhausted, and I determined to make the experiment whether they might not be literally scouted out of their hiding-places. I first rubbed the bedstead with elder flowers, but, to my cost, the perverse inhabitants did not dislike the scent; for although I killed all that I saw at the time, in two weeks after they were as numerous as ever. Walking in the garden the same day, I accidentally touched a tomato vine, the smell of which is peculiarly nauseous to me; the thought suddenly occurred that it might be equally so to my enemies. I immediately went to work, and had the bedsteads thoroughly rubbed with the green vine. I have not since discovered any of my tormentors. I inform you of this, as I wish others would try if the tomato vine will always have the effect I suppose it had in this case.—*A Farmer's Wife.*

TO PREVENT FLEAS INFESTING ROOMS OR BEDS.

Take a few branches of pennyroyal, and hang it up or lay it on the bed, or carry a few sprigs in the pocket, and the flea will never make its appearance. This simple remedy has never failed of the desired effect.

A CURE FOR THE RED ANTS.

The evils of this little visitant are well known to

perhaps every housewife, and perhaps nothing would more exhilarate the domestic circle than the discovery of a remedy for the red ants. Such discovery I have made, and wish you to communicate to the public through your useful paper. Common salt is a complete barrier to the approach of the red ant. Let the salt be so placed, that they cannot approach the place from which you wish to exclude them, without passing over it, and the remedy is complete. For instance, if you wish to exclude them from the cellar, cupboard, or any moveable cupboard, if it has no legs, make artificial legs to your cupboard; then provide something suitable to hold a pint of salt, in which place the legs of the cupboard, and set it free from everything else, so that nothing can creep on to it without passing over the salt, and the remedy is complete.

TO DESTROY FLIES.

White arsenic, one drachm; water one pint; dissolve by boiling, and sweeten with molasses.

ANOTHER.—Half a spoonful of ground black pepper, one teaspoonful of brown sugar, one tablespoonful of cream, mixed well together, and placed on a plate, will attract and destroy flies without any danger of poisoning children.

A SIMPLE WAY OF PREVENTING FLIES FROM SITTING ON PICTURES, OR ANY OTHER FURNITURE.

Let a large bunch of leeks soak for five or six days in a pailful of water, and wash your pictures or any piece of furniture, with it. The flies will never come near anything so washed. This secret is very important and well experienced.

TO DESTROY COCKROACHES.

Preserve a moderate quantity of pokeroot, boil it in

water until the juice is extracted, and mingle the liquor with good molasses; spread the liquor in platters or soup plates in the kitchen, pantry, or closet, wash-house, or whatever apartment is infested by them, and the enemy will be found slain in heaps by the following morning. A gentleman, to whom we are indebted for this information, states that he slaughtered five hundred and seventy-five cockroaches in a single night, by means of the pokeroot and molasses, and that root which had been boiled being thrown into a closet thickly infested by the enemy, the place was quitted by them entirely in a few days, great numbers being left dead upon the field.

TO CLEAN FLINT GLASS BOTTLES, DECANTERS, ETC.

Roll up, in small pieces, some whited, brown, or blotting paper, then wet and soap the same; put them into the vessel with a little warm water; shake them well for a few minutes, then rinse with clean water, and it will be as bright and clear as when new from the shops.

METHOD FOR CLEANING FINE BLOCK TIN DISH COVERS, PATENT PEWTER, ETC.

Where the polish has gone off, let the articles be rubbed over the outside with a little sweet oil on a piece of soft linen cloth, then clean it off with dry pure whiting, quite free from sand, on linen cloths, which will make them look as well as when new. The insides should be rubbed with rags moistened in wet whiting, but without a drop of oil: always wiping these articles dry when brought from the table; and keeping them free from steam or other dampness, greatly diminishes the trouble of cleaning them.

CEMENT FOR MENDING BROKEN CROCKERY, CHINA, OR GLASS WARE.

Mix half a pint of skimmed milk with an equal quantity of vinegar, so as to coagulate the milk. Separate the curd from the whey, and mix the former with whites of four or five eggs, after beating them up well. The mixture of these two substances being complete, add sifted quicklime, and make the whole into a thick paste of the consistence of putty. If this be carefully applied to broken bodies, or to fissures of any kind, and dried properly, it resists fire and water.

ANOTHER.—Pound burned oyster shells, sift the powder through a very fine sieve, and grind it on a painter's stone till reduced to the finest powder; then take the whites of several eggs, according to the quantity of powder, beat them well, and having mixed them with the powder, form the whole into a kind of paste; join the pieces of china or glass and press them together for seven or eight minutes, and the united parts will stand heat and water, and will not come apart if they should fall on the ground.

CHINESE METHOD OF MENDING CHINA.

Take a piece of flint glass, beat it to a fine powder, and grind it with the white of an egg, and it joins without riveting, so that no art can break it in the same place. You are to observe that the composition is to be ground extremely fine on a painter's stone.

HOW TO GET A TIGHT RING OFF A FINGER.

Thread a needle, flat in the eye, with a strong thread, pass the head of the needle, with care, under the ring, and pull the thread through a few inches towards the hand; wrap the long end of the thread tightly round the finger, regularly all down to the nail, to reduce its size. Then lay hold of the short end and unwind it. The thread passing against the ring, will gradually remove it from the finger. This never failing method will remove the tightest ring without difficulty, however much swollen the finger may be.

TO EXTRACT A GLASS STOPPER.

Take a large strip of wool; pass it once around the neck of the bottle; attach one end of this to a board, or some fixed object; hold the other, and then seesaw the bottle along it. The friction will soon heat the neck of the bottle, and by the heat the neck will expand sufficiently to allow of the stopper being extracted.

TO REMOVE PANES OF GLASS.

Put soft soap on the putty for a few hours, and it becomes as soft as if just put on, though the putty had become as hard as a stone.

PASTE.

Putting acetate or sugar of lead into it, instead of the old way of mixing it with alum, keeps it from moulding, clear, and quite moist for months together.

TO CLEAN PAINT THAT IS NOT VARNISHED.

Put upon a plate some of the best whiting; have ready some clear warm water, and a piece of flannel, which dip into the water, and squeeze nearly dry; then take as much whiting as will adhere to it; apply it to the paint, when a little rubbing will instantly remove any dirt or grease. Wash well off with water, and rub it dry with a soft cloth. Paint thus cleansed looks equal to new, and without doing the least injury to the most delicate colour. It will preserve the paint much longer than if cleaned with soap, and it does not require more than half the time usually occupied in cleaning.

A WASH TO CLEAN PICTURES.

Make a ley with clear water and wood ashes; in this dip a sponge, and rub the pictures over, and it cleanses it perfectly. The same may be done with chamber ley only; or otherwise, with white wine; and it will have the same effect.

A SECRET TO REVIVE OLD WRITINGS, WHICH ARE ALMOST DEFACED.

Boil gall-nuts into wine; then steeping a sponge into that liquor, and passing it on the lines of the old writing, all the letters which were almost undecipherable will appear as fresh as newly done.

TO PREVENT MOULDING IN BOOKS, INK, PASTE, AND LEATHER.

Collectors of books will not be sorry to learn that a few drops of oil of lavender will ensure their libraries from this pest. A single drop of the same oil will prevent a pint of ink from moulding any length of time. Paste may be kept from mould entirely by its addition; and leather is also effectually secured from injury by the same agency.

TO CLEAN KNIVES AND FORKS.

Procure a smooth board, cover it with leather; melt a sufficient quantity of mutten suet, and put it hot upon the leather with a piece of flannel. Then take two pieces of soft Bath brick, and rub them one against the other over the leather till it is covered with the powder, which rub in until no grease comes through when a knife is passed over the leather, which may be easily known by the knife's keeping its polish.

TO KEEP UP SASH WINDOWS.

This is performed by means of cork, in the simplest manner, and with scarcely any expense. Bore three or four holes in the sides of the sash, into which insert common bottle corks, projecting about the sixteenth part of an inch. These will press against the frames, along the usual grooves, and by their elasticity support the sash at any height which may be required.

COMPOSITION FOR RAZORS.

Common candle snuff, clear of grit, spread on a razor strap, produces the best edge, in the shortest time, of anything ever tried. The coat should be spread with a knife, not too thick, and will last several months; first rub the strap with a little clean tallow.

WOOD POLISHING.

The Persians have introduced an entirely new mode of polishing, which is to wood precisely what plating is to metal. Water may be spilled on it without staining, and it resists scratching the same as marble. The receipt for making it as follows:—

To one pint of spirits of wine, add half an ounce of gum shellac, half an ounce of gum sandrick, placing it over a gentle heat, frequently agitating it until the gums are dissolved, when it is fit for use.

Make a roller of list, put a little of the polish upon it, and cover that with a soft linen rag, which must be slightly touched with cold drawn linseed oil. Rub them in the wood, in a circular direction, not covering too large a space at a time, till the pores are sufficiently filled up. After this, rub in the same manner spirits of wine with a small portion of the polish added to it, and a most brilliant polish will be produced. If the outside has been previously polished with wax, it will be necessary to clean it off with glass paper.—*Western Farmer.*

POLISH FOR DINING TABLES.

Rub them with cold drawn linseed oil, thus :—Put a little in the middle of a table, and then with a piece of linen (never use woollen) cloth, rub it well all over the table ; then take another piece of linen, and rub it for ten minutes ; then rub it quite dry with another cloth. This must be done every day for several months, when you will find your mahogany acquire a permanent and beautiful lustre, unattainable by any other means, and equal to the finest French polish ; and if the table is covered with the table cloth only, the hottest dishes will make no impression upon it. When once this polish is produced, it will only require dry rubbing with a linen cloth for about ten minutes twice in a week to preserve it in the highest perfection.

COMPOSITION FOR MAKING COMMON WOOD RESEMBLE MAHOGANY.

It has been contrived to render any species of wood, of a close grain, so nearly to resemble mahogany in the nature, density and polish, that the most accurate judges are incapable of distinguishing between this happy imitation and the native produce. The first operation, as now practised in France, is to plane the surface so as to render it perfectly smooth ; the wood is then to be rubbed with diluted nitrous acid, which prepares it for the materials subsequently to be applied. Afterward one ounce and a half of dragon's blood, dissolved in a pint of spirits of wine, and one-third of that quantity of carbonate of soda, are to be mixed together and filtered, and the liquid in this state is to be rubbed, or rather laid upon the wood with a soft brush. This process is repeated, with very little alteration; and in a short interval afterward the wood possesses the external appearance of mahogany; when this application has been properly made, the surface will resemble an artificial mirror: but if the polish become less brilliant, by rubbing it with a little cold drawn linseed oil the wood will be restored to its former brilliancy.

USEFUL COMPOSITION.

To prevent friction, and facilitate the running of machinery, the best thing in use is said to be grease, eight parts, to two parts of black lead, intimately mixed.

TO PREVENT THE SMOKING OF A LAMP.

Soak the wick in strong vinegar, and dry it well before you use it; it will then burn both sweet and pleasant, and give much satisfaction for the trifling trouble in preparing it.

SMOKY CHIMNEYS.

It has been clearly demonstrated by science and practical experiments that this great drawback upon domestic comfort is remedied by an unerring and simple process, viz., a slight but continued enlargement, commencing at the bottom of the flue, and extending to the top. This is sure to produce a draught, and it is presumed that in most instances of defective chimneys, inattention to this simple rule, in the original construction, would be found the cause of the evil.

A VALUABLE MORTAR TO PREVENT SOOT FROM ACCUMULATING IN CHIMNEYS.

Instead of plastering the inside of chimneys in the

usual way, take mortar made with one peck of salt to each bushel of lime, adding as much sand and lime as will render it fit to work, and then lay on a thick coat. If the chimney has no offsets for the soot to lodge on, it will continue perfectly clear and free from all danger of taking fire. The writer of this has tried the experiment, and after three years constant use of a chimney plastered as above directed he could never obtain a quart of soot, though he several times employed a sweeper to scrape it from top to bottom.

A COMPOSITION TO DEFEND THE ROOF OF A HOUSE FROM THE WEATHER AND FIRE.

Take one measure of fine sand, two measures of wood ashes well sifted, three of slackened lime ground up with oil, laid on with a painter's brush—first coat thin, and second thick. I painted on a board with this mixture, and it adheres so strongly to the board that it resists an iron tool; and put thick on a shingle resists the operation of fire. I used only a part of the mixture; what remains in an iron pot water has lain on for some time, without penetrating the substance, which is as hard as a stone.

COMPOSITION FOR PRESERVING FARMERS' UTENSILS.

Take three-fourths of a pound of resin in an iron kettle, with three gallons of train oil, and three or four rolls of brimstone; when they are melted and become thin, add as much Spanish brown, or any other color you choose, ground up in oil in the usual way, as will give the color you desire; then lay on a thin coat with a brush, and when dry lay on another. This will preserve barrows, ploughs, carts, wagons, yokes, gate posts, weather boards, shingles, &c., many years from the effects of the weather.

ON THE PRESERVATION OF HARNESS.

Allow me to recommend the following method of preserving leather, harness, and traces, engine hose, boots, and shoes, cording, cart and wagon covers, stack cloths, &c., in the most effectual manner. Take of neatsfoot oil one quart; beeswax, cut small, one ounce; oil of tar half a pound; and after simmering the neatsfoot oil and wax a little in a pipkin, the oil of tar must be added; when, after a gentle simmering again for a few minutes, stirring it the whole time with a stick, the mixture will be finished. At the same time, if an ounce of naptha were added, it would be a considerable improvement: it is used precisely as oil would be applied, and where it may be required to soften old and hardened leather, a washing, or sponging with hot water first, is advisable, and the liquid should be driven in before the fire. Leather, or cordage, dressed with this liquid, never rots, hardens, grows mouldy, nor perishes with blacking.

It is likewise a complete destroyer of scabbiness in sheep, or other animals. I gave the form about seven years back to a person who made a benefit of its sale in town, and afterward, contrary to a pledge given me, sold the same to two people, who now retail a very inferior composition. As to the expense, one application of this fluid is superior to four or five of oil. Where the rendering leather water-proof is desirable, the ounce of naptha proposed to be added should have a drachm of Indian rubber dissolved in it; for it should be remembered that those things which give suppleness to leather, open its pores, whereas to make it water-proof, the closing up by astringent applications, or filling them up by waxy, or gummy ones, is indispensable. It is, perhaps, right to add, that nap-

that is highly inflammable, and therefore should be kept from the fire and candle, and added after the mixture is taken from the fire.

A COMPOSITION FOR PRESERVING BOOTS AND SHOES.

The receipt is as follows, and is to be used for the "uppers" only :—one half pint neatsfoot oil, one ounce beeswax, one ounce spirits turpentine, one ounce tar, one half ounce Burgundy pitch, to be slowly melted together and well incorporated by stirring, taking care not to set the mass on fire, as the articles are all highly inflammable. The boots being damp, the composition is to be spread on with a small brush, taking care to cover the seams well, and then be allowed to dry; the application to be renewed until the leather is saturated.

The above is for the "upper leather"—for the soles, tar alone is the best application, to be put on while hot, the boots also having been by the fire, so that the soles are quite warm; if there is no grease or other foreign matter on the soles, three or four, or sometimes more, coats will sink into the leather; it must also be used until the soles are completely saturated. The trouble of preparing boots after the above directions is very trifling, and any one once having tried it, and experienced the comfort of being all day in the snow and slush without having wet feet, will never fail to continue the use of it.

BLACKING,

Which, when on the boots or shoes, can be rubbed with a cambric handkerchief without soiling it in the least, and will assume the same lustre after being plunged in water as before. Quarter of a pound of ivory black, one ounce of sweet oil, one ounce spirits of lavender, one ounce oil of vitriol, two ounces sugar candy, three pints best vinegar, or stale beer, and juice of two lemons.

Note.—The ivory black and sweet oil to be well mixed in a mortar, the sugar candy to be pounded, the vitriol to be put in a glass of water, and let stand till cold. The spirits of lavender and oil of vitriol not to be put in until all the other ingredients have been well mixed.

Another.—The following are said to be the materials of which Day and Martin's blacking is made:—

To one pound of ivory black, in which has been mixed half an ounce of oil of vitriol and one ounce of sweet oil, add one pound of pulverized loaf sugar; mix the whole with a gallon of vinegar and let it stand three days, when it is fit for use.

It should be stirred often, and kept from the air to prevent evaporation. The cost of a gallon of this blacking is seventy-five cents, and is retailed at the stores for four dollars.

TO PREVENT SHOES FROM TAKING IN WATER.

One pint of drying oil, two ounces of yellow wax, two ounces of turpentine, half an ounce Burgundy pitch, melted carefully over a slow fire. If new boots or shoes are rubbed carefully with this mixture, either in the sunshine or at some distance from the fire, with a sponge or soft brush, and the operation is repeated as often as they become dry, till the leather is fully saturated, they will be impervious to the wet, and will wear much longer, as well as acquiring a softness and pliability that will prevent the leather from ever shrivelling.

Note.—Shoes or boots prepared as above ought not

to be worn until perfectly dry and elastic, otherwise their durability would rather be prevented than increased.

JAPAN COPAL VARNISH.

The following receipt and directions for manufacturing and using this varnish, we believe originated in Italy. The secret of the process was made known in the United States by an Italian, whose knowledge of the art has been a source of considerable profit to himself. The materials and proportions used are as follows:

One ounce gum copal, one ounce gum Arabic, one ounce draganda (tragacanth), four ounces gum shellac, and one quarter of an ounce of gum myrrh; pound it fine, and put it in a quart of alcohol; let it stand for half an hour: after that, your composition is fit for use.

For colouring red, one quarter of an ounce of Sanders yellow, one quarter of a pound of turmeric. Black, one quarter of an ounce of lamp-black.

Wood may be coloured any colour, and when dry, this varnish will give it the gloss.

The best material for black colour is the oil varnish, which may be obtained at any drug store. To prepare the work for varnishing, oil it completely with linseed oil, put on with a sponge.

How to apply the Varnish.—Absorb the varnish with a sponge, a sufficient quantity to varnish the piece of work which is to be finished (three or four table spoonsful is sufficient for a sideboard), over which you must put a cotton or linen cloth; then apply to the cloth a little portion of linseed oil, which may be frequently repeated while varnishing. The varnish dries as it is applied to the work, and at the same time gives the tint or shade required, if the colouring material is mixed with it.

The varnish may be mixed with the colouring material, and the varnish and colouring all done at the same time, or the colouring may be given first; after which the varnish may be applied. If the varnish and colouring is to be performed at the same time, a sufficient quantity of varnish and colouring matter must be mixed together to varnish the work to be finished. If, however, it is desirable to varnish and colour separately, the colour should be laid on first, and when dry the varnish may be laid on as above directed.

TO MAKE JAPANESE CEMENT, OR RICE GLUE.

This elegant cement is made by mixing rice flour intimately with cold water, and then gently boiling it. It is beautifully white, and dries almost transparent. Papers pasted together by means of this cement will sooner separate in their own substance than at the joining, which makes it extremely useful in the preparation of curious paper articles, as tea trays, ladies' dressing-boxes, and other articles which require layers of paper to be cemented together. It is in every respect preferable to common paste made with wheat flour, for almost every purpose to which that article is usually applied. It answers in particular, for pasting into books the copies of writings taken off by copying machines or insized silver paper. With this composition, made with a comparatively small quantity of water, that it may have the consistence similar to plastic clay, models, busts, stays, and the like may be formed when dry. The articles made of it are susceptible of a very high polish. They are also very durable.

TO MAKE A BEAUTIFUL AND LASTING WHITEWASH.

Take a quarter of a peck of unslacked lime, pour on it a kettle of boiling water; while the lime is slacking add half a gallon of stale chamber ley; when the lime is perfectly slacked, dilute it with water to the proper consistence, and add to this mixture one quarter of an ounce of Prussian blue. This will give you a beautiful and lasting wash, that will neither peel off nor turn yellow, and will look nearly as well as white paint. By increasing the quantity of blue, you may make either a pale or a dark blue, as best suits your taste: or, if you prefer it, by adding yellow or red ochre, you may impart either of these tints to your wash.

TO MAKE A BRILLIANT STUCCO WHITEWASH FOR BUILDINGS, INSIDE OR OUT.

Add one quarter of a pound of whiting, or burned alum pulverized, one pound of loaf sugar, three quarts of rice flour made into a thin and well boiled paste, one pound of the cleanest glue dissolved as cabinetmakers do. This mixture may be put on cold within doors, but hot outside. This preparation will be as brilliant as plaster of Paris, and retain its brilliancy for many years. The east end of the President's house is washed with it.

TO MAKE A CHEAP PAINT, OR WHITEWASH.

Take two quarts of skimmed milk, two ounces of fresh slacked lime, and five pounds of whiting. Put the lime into a stone vessel, pour upon it a sufficient quantity of milk to make a mixture resembling cream, then add the remainder of the milk. When this is done, crumble and spread the whiting on the surface of the fluid, in which it will gradually sink. It must, after all the whiting has been precipitated, be well stirred, or ground as you would other paint, when it will be fit for use. By the addition of any colouring matter, you may make it to suit your fancy. It should be put on with a paint brush, and when dry a second coat should be given. The quantity above mentioned is sufficient for twenty-seven yards.

ANOTHER.—Take one bushel of unslacked lime, and slack it with cold water; when well slacked, add to it 20 lbs. of Spanish whiting, 17 lbs. of salt, and 12 lbs. of sugar. Strain this mixture through a wire sieve, and it will be fit for use after reducing it with cold water. This is intended for the outside of a building, where it is exposed to all weather. In order to give a good colour, three coats are necessary on brick, and two on wood. It may be laid on with a whitewash brush. Each coat must have a sufficient time to dry before the next is applied. For painting inside walls take as before, one bushel of unslacked lime, 3 lbs. of sugar, 5 lbs. of salt, and prepare as above, and apply with a brush. It is well calculated to preserve brick walls; and is far preferable to oil paint. This paint will preserve rough boards longer than they would be from dressing them and covering them with oil paint. You can make any colour you please. For straw colour use yellow ochre instead of whiting; for lemon colour, ochre and chrome yellow; for lead and slate colour, lampblack; for blue, indigo; for green, chrome green. These different kinds of paints will not cost one fourth as much as oil paints, including the putting on.

A CHEAP WHITE PAINT.

One pound of unslacked lime, one pound of Spanish whiting, one gallon of sweet milk, one gallon of flax-seed oil, one tablespoonful of salt; pour on the lime sufficient water to slack it, and while the lime is slacking pour in the oil so as to cook it thin; add the whiting and salt, then pour on the milk and stir it well.

A CHEAP GREEN PAINT.

Take four pounds of Roman vitriol, and pour upon it a tea-kettle full of boiling water: when the vitriol is dissolved add two pounds of pearlash, and stir the mixture well with a stick until the effervescence ceases; then add a quarter of a pound of pulverized yellow arsenic, and stir the whole together. Lay it on with a paint brush, and if the wall has not been painted, two or three coats will be necessary. If a pea green be required, put on less, and if an apple green, more of the yellow arsenic.

The cost of this paint is less than one-fourth of oil colour, and the beauty far superior.—*Yankee Farmer.*

PERMANENT INK FOR MARKING LINEN.

This useful ink is composed of nitrate of silver (lunar caustic) and tincture, or infusion of galls, in the proportions of one drachm of the former in a dry state, to two drachms of the latter. The linen, cotton, or commodity, must be first soaked in the following liquid, viz.: salt of tartar, one ounce, dissolved in one ounce and a half of water, and must be perfectly dry before any attempt is made to write upon it.

MARKING OR DURABLE INK.

Take six and a quarter cents worth of lunar caustic, and having put it into an ounce phial full of vinegar, cork it tight and hang it in the sun. In a couple of days it will be fit for use. To make the preparation for the above, take a lump of pearlash of the size of a chestnut and dissolve it in a gill of rain water. The part of the muslin or linen to be written upon, is to be wet with the preparation, and dried and glazed with a warm flat iron : immediately after which, it is ready for marking.

TO MAKE BLACK INK.

In three pints of vinegar, let three ounces of gall-nuts, one ounce powdered logwood, and one ounce green vitriol, be steeped half an hour ; then add one half ounce gum-arabic, and when the gum is dissolved, pass the whole mixture through a hair sieve.

IMPROVED COMPOSITION OF BLACK WRITING INK.

Take a gallon of soft water, and boil in it one pound of chips of logwood for about half an hour; then take the decoction from the fire, and pour it from off the chips, while boiling hot, on a pound of the best Aleppo galls, reduced to a fine powder, and two ounces of pomegranate peels ; put into a proper vessel. After having stirred them well together with a wooden spoon or ladle for some time, place them in the sunshine in summer, or within the warmth of the fire if in winter, for three or four days, stirring the mixture as often as may be convenient ; at the end of that time, add half a pound of green vitriol, powdered, and let the mixture remain four or five days more, stirring it frequently, and then add further four ounces gum arabic dissolved in a quart of boiling water ; and after giving the ink some time to settle, strain it off from the dregs, and keep it well stopped for use.

If the ink be desired to shine more, the proportion of the pomegranate peel must be increased.

In order to secure this ink from growing mouldy, a quarter of a pint of spirits of wine may be added, but to prevent its containing any acid which may injure the ink, a little salt of tartar or pearlash should be added previously, and the spirits poured off from it.

FOR MAKING RED INK.

Infuse four ounces of ground Brazil wood in one quart of vinegar for three days, then heat it to the boiling point, and keep it for an hour at that temperature; after which it must be filtrated. While hot, dissolve in it one third of an ounce of gum arabic, and the same quantity of sugar, and of alum; allow it to cool, and put it into bottles well stopped. An ink of a still more beautiful shade may be made with a decoction of cochineal, to which ammonia is to be added.

HOW TO PREPARE PRINTER'S INK.

1. Take one pound of common turpentine, made with the sandarak of the ancients, which is nothing else but juniper and linseed oil. Add to it one ounce of resin black, which is the smoke of it, and a sufficient quantity of oil of nuts.

2. Set this composition on the fire, and boil it to a good consistence. Such is the whole secret. Observe, however, that in the summer it must boil a little more, and a little less in winter. For in the summer the ink must be thicker, and thinner in the winter, because the heat makes it more fluid. In which case it is therefore proper to boil it a little more, or to diminish the quantity of oil allowed in the proportion to that of the turpentine.

FOR STOPPING A LEAK IN A CASK.

The best thing for stopping a leak in a cask is whiting beaten up with common yellow soap. If this mixture be well rubbed into the leak, it will be found to stop it after everything else has failed.

TO PRESERVE NAILS FROM RUSTING.

Take cut nails, and heat them pretty hot in a fire-shovel over the fire, but not red hot, and then drop them into a glazed vessel containing train oil. They absorb a good deal of oil, and when thus prepared, never become rusty, and will last many years. Hinges and screws that are exposed to the weather would do well to be treated in the same way. Would not the preparation of cut or wrought nails used in making board fences, or in any place where there is considerable exposure to the weather, in the manner recommended above, be a decided improvement?

GREASE FOR WHEEL AXLES.

It is more than twenty years since we employed the following composition, which was revealed to us as a great secret, and for which money had been usually demanded :—Thicken half a pint of melted grease with black lead in powder, having previously thrown in and melted a lump of beeswax of the size of a small hickory nut. Apply it to the hubs and axles before it hardens. By using this composition we have on various occasions driven our carriage two or three hundred miles without once greasing it after we started; and subsequent examinations have satisfied us that no attention of the kind is necessary in such journeys. In warm weather we use tallow instead of soft grease. Black lead is sometimes gritty, that is, it contains sand, and such should be rejected. If tar has been previously applied to the hubs and axles, it ought to be carefully removed before the composition is applied; and until the pores of the wood become filled with the composition, it may escape from the boxes in that way, and render frequent examinations for the first few weeks necessary.

Genesee Farmer.

BROWNING STEEL OR IRON.

Some easy method of browning or forming a permanent oxyde on iron or steel, has long been a desideratum with artists on those metals; and from the difficulty of the method as usually conducted, and its being considered an important secret, it has generally been confined to gun barrels, &c. After a long series of experiments, Mr. Ettrich has discovered, and made known in a foreign journal, a process of procuring a permanent oxyde, and then giving it a dark brown or black colour. The iron or steel of a rifle barrel, for instance, must be well smothered and polished, and all greasiness removed by chalk before browning commences. Then mix one part of nitric acid with one hundred parts of water, and, moistening a rag in this, apply it to the barrel. It is material that the rag should only be moistened, for if instead of damping the iron, the fluid streams over it, the browning will be imperfect and irregular. The barrel, after being wet, should be placed in a window on which the sun shines, for an hour or more; and when this process has been twice or thrice repeated, the superfluous rust must be removed by a scratch brush consisting of a quantity of fine wire tied up into a bundle. This process being repeated eight or ten times, the barrel will have acquired as perfect a brown as is usually given by gunsmiths; but to do away the rusty appearance that remains on the iron, it is browned, or blacked, by dissolving one grain of nitrate of silver in five hundred of water, and applying this solution in the same way as the acid. The number of repetitions of nitrate of silver water will depend on the shade of blackness required, but from one to five will be sufficient: at each wetting with the nitrate, the barrel should be placed in the sunshine, to ensure a dark colour. The last process is to apply the scratch freely, though lightly, and then polish the whole down by beeswax. Mr. Ettrich found by experiment, after becoming acquainted with the process used by the trade, that his system of operation produced a much finer and darker brown than could be given by theirs, and is decidedly more simple and easy in being carried into effect.

PIG TROUGHS.

Take two pieces of board or plank, of the length that you wish your trough; put two of their edges together at right angles, thus V, and nail them strong; then take two pieces, something longer than the trough is wide, and nail upon the ends; then take some clay mortar and fill up the chinks to prevent its leaking, and it is done. The food settles down in the bottom of the trough, and the pig will lay his sharp under jaw into it completely, while the long ends prevent its being upset so easily as the old kind. Anybody who can saw a board off, or drive a nail, can make one. If you have no trough for your pig, just try your hand at making one on this plan.

Genesee Farmer.

FENCE POSTS.

An excellent method of rendering these durable in the ground consists, 1st. In peeling the posts, and in sawing and splitting them, if too large. 2d. In sticking them up under cover, at least one entire summer; and, 3d. In coating with hot tar about three feet of the butt ends, which are to be inserted in the ground; after which they are ready for use. We have no doubt that the advantages of this mode of preparation will more than remunerate for labour and expense. Our reasons for this belief are briefly as follows :—The sap of all non-resinous trees will ferment in the presence of heat and moisture, and cause the decay of the wood. To prevent this natural consequence, the first object should be, where a tree is filled, to expel the sap from the pores of the wood. This is done by peeling, splitting, sawing, or hewing, and exposing the wood to the drying influence of the sun, or at least of the air. The process is facilitated, too, by immersing the wood in water for a time, which liquefies the sap, and favours its expulsion. And when the moisture has been expelled, the next object is to keep it out by paint, tar, or charring. In the mode recommended above, the mixture is expelled by the peeling, sawing, and summer drying; and its return is prevented by the coating of tar. The retention of the bark upon timber is particularly prejudicial, not only in preventing evaporation, but affording shelter to various species of the borer, which under its cover carry on their depredations upon the timber. We have seen fine logs nearly destroyed in a summer by worms, where the bark had been left on; while those which had been peeled remained uninjured. The best timber is obtained from trees which have stood in summer, or a year, after they have been girdled and peeled.

ANOTHER.—The durability of posts used in making fences is a matter of great importance to farmers, and will continue so as long as the present system of fencing is continued. We are informed that the Shakers of Union Village have been in the habit of making oak posts as durable as locnst, by a very simple and easy process. This is merely to bore a hole in that part of the post which will be just at the surface of the earth, with such a slope as will carry it just below the surface, and fill it with salt. This, it is said, will preserve the timber from decaying for a long time; and, from the knowledge we have of the influence of salt in preserving ship timber, when treated in a similar manner, we have no doubt of its being an excellent method.—*American Farmer*.

MEASURING CORN.

Having previously levelled the corn in the house, so that it will be of equal depth throughout, ascertain the length, depth, and breadth of the bulk; multiply these dimensions together, and their products by four; then cut off one figure from the right of the last product: this will give so many bushels, and decimal bushels of shelled corn. If it be required to find the quantity of corn in the ears, substitute 8 for 4, and cut off one figure as before.

Example.—In a bulk of corn in the ears, measuring twelve feet long, eleven feet broad, and six feet deep, there will be 316 bushels and eight-tenths of a bushel of shelled corn; or 633 bushels of ears as follows.

```
          12              12
          11              11
         ———             ———
         132             132
           6               6
         ———             ———
         792             792
           4               8
         ———             ———
Shell corn, 316.8        633.6 ears.
```

The decimal 4 is used when the object is to find the quantity in shelled corn, because that decimal is half of the decimal, and it requires two bushels of ears to make one of shelled corn. In using these rules, a half bushel should be added for every hundred, that amount of error resulting from the substitution of the decimals.

TO CALCULATE INTEREST.

A short and simple method of calculating interest at six per cent. per annum.

Rule.—Multiply the principal by half the number of months.

Example.—What is the interest of forty dollars for twelve months?

$40 the principal.
6 half the number of months.
───────
$2.40 answer.

Example.—What is the interest of forty dollars for seven months?

$40
3-1-2
───────
1.20
20
───────
$1.40 *answer.*

EFFECTUAL METHOD OF KILLING WASPS.

When a wasp's nest is found, take about half a pint of tar in a pitch ladle, and run part of it into a hole where the nest is; put the remainder of the tar round about the mouth of the hole, and the job is done. All the wasps that are in the nest are caught in their attempt to come out, and those that are out are caught in their attempt to go in, so that none escape. If the nest should be in a place where the tar will soon get dry, it may perhaps be better to put a little more tar round the hole the following day, as in general there are a great many of them which are out all night, and when the tar is dry it will not catch them. It is not necessary to dig out the nest, and the tar may be applied at any time of the day, even when the wasps are most busy.

NOTE.—Should the wasps build their nests any place out of the ground, they might easily be destroyed by smoking them well with brimstone after night.

IMPORTANT DISCOVERY; OR, HOW TO KILL CROWS WITH NEW-ENGLAND RUM.

At length the ingenuity, or good luck of this ingenious and lucky age, has discovered one valuable use to which ardent spirits can be applied, viz., the clearing of our cornfields of crows. The first experiments have proved quite successful, and are reported in the Wiscasset Citizen as follows :

Some lads in a neighbouring town, highly delighted with the new law giving a bounty of eight cents on crows, but thinking the bounty too low for powder and shot, took the following method of testing the law as well as the profits, by killing with something more sure and deadly in its effects than powder and shot, viz., New-England rum! They soaked some corn in a quantity of rum, until it was saturated therewith, and then spread it in a cornfield infested with crows. The boys were in ambuscade. The crows came on as usual by platoons, and commenced devouring the corn. In a few moments the young rogues had the satisfaction of seeing their sagacious foe so completely corned, to use their own phrase, as to tumble about in high snuff. They cautiously approached; but what was their surprise as they drew nigh to find them as drunk as David's sow, and in this situation they knocked a number of them in the head in one forenoon.

TO PREVENT CROWS FROM PULLING UP CORN.

Soak seed corn in a solution of Glauber salts, from twenty-four to forty-eight hours before planting, and no living animal, with the sense of taste, will eat it. This method of preventing crows from destroying corn was accidentally discovered by John B. Swasey, Esq., of Meredith, N. H., several years since. He directed his hired man to soak a quantity of seed corn preparatory to planting, in a solution of saltpetre. By mistake Glauber salts were taken for nitre; the mistake was not discovered, until it was nearly all planted; the piece of ground was finished with dry corn. That part of the piece planted with soaked corn remained undisturbed; while the dry corn was nearly all destroyed by crows, blackbirds, and squirrels.

SCARE-CROWS.

The best scare-crows we have ever used, were bright sheets of tin suspended from poles, by wires; the poles of sufficient height, and in sufficient numbers, to be seen all over the field. Four or six, if judiciously placed, will effectually answer for a field of fifty acres. Our mode of fixing them was this; we cut a pole of sufficient height, trimmed off all the limbs but the upper ones; to the end of this limb, we attached by a strong flexible wire, a sheet of tin, and planted the pole thus provided firmly in the ground on the destined spot. The limb left at the top, should project horizontally far enough to allow full play to the tin. Thus attached, the slightest breeze gives motion to the tin, and consequently causes a reflection so sudden as to effectually frighten off crows, or other birds addicted to picking up the corn. Three years successful use of such scare-crows justify us in recommending them to our brethren.

METHOD OF DESTROYING WOLVES AND CROWS.

If you think the following information would be of any service to any of your subscribers, it is at their service. I have a mountain farm that would afford excellent pasture for sheep, but it was so infested with wolves, that it would have been very hazardous to risk them there. In order to destroy them, we took an old horse, and bled him in such a way as to make a train of blood for about five miles; we then killed him; and having stuck a great many holes in him, put about a grain of strychnine into each hole. I also removed the skin off one hip and thigh, where most of the poison was put. The skin was dragged four or five miles, coming back again to the horse; all the wolves in the neighborhood were in this way brought by the trails to the horse. Several dead ones were found near the horse; and they have been scarce in that neighborhood since.

I have also killed all the crows on my farm in the same way. I took a quarter of veal, and having cut up a portion of it into small pieces, and mixed strychnine with them, I stuck many holes in the meat, and put one of these small pieces in each place. I also sprinkled strychnine over the meat, and then put the veal in a place where the dogs could not get to it, and where the crows resorted; and in a few days there was not a crow to be seen on my farm, except dead ones, which could be picked up all over the place.

For four or five years I have killed my crows in the month of April, shortly after they build their nests and become stationary, and am not troubled with them any more, until they begin to gather in flocks in the fall of the year.

If a dog should by accident get poisoned with strychnine or nux vomica, an emetic of tartar will cure him. It will require a teaspoonful or more to operate.

ESTIMATING THE WEIGHT OF CATTLE.

In a country like ours, where great numbers of cattle are annually bought and sold, under circumstances that forbid the ascertaining their weight with positive accuracy, it must be desirable that some general rules, approximating to exactness, should be known, in order to prevent all ground of mistake or collision on the part of the interested individuals. In England, two or three tables have been constructed by different individuals, founded on the length and girth of the animal, at certain points, and based on a vast number of experiments, most carefully made. To illustrate this matter, we have copied from an English work the figure and tables, as follows.

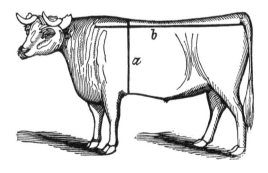

Girth.	Length.	Renton's Table.	Cary's Guage
feet. in.	feet. in.	stone. lb.	stone. lb
5 0	3 6	21 0	21 0
	4 0	24 0	24 0
5 6	3 9	27 1	27 0
	4 0	34 4	34 7
6 0	4 6	38 8	38 11
	5 0	43 1	43 0
6 6	4 6	45 9	45 7
	4 9	48 0	48 0
7 0	5 6	64 6	64 7
	6 0	70 5	70 3
8 0	6 6	99 8	99 12
	7 0	107 5	107 6

In taking the girth and length of an animal, the manner is as follows :—The girth is taken by passing a line just behind the shoulder blade, and under the fore legs (see line on the figure): this gives the circumference of the animal. The length is taken along the back, from the foremost corner of the blade-bone of the shoulder, in a straight line, to the hindmost point of the rump, or to that bone of the tail that plumbs the line with the hinder part of the buttock. These lines are then measured by the foot rule, and the weight can readily be calculated from the tables. Some slight difference of weight may be traced in the tables, and also in another one, calculated by M. Derment: but the agreement is sufficiently close to show that no material error can exist. The tables, according to the English mode of reckoning, are calculated upon the stone of fourteen pounds, avoirdupois; thus, if the girth is six feet, and the length five feet, the weight will be forty-three stone, one pound, or six hundred and three pounds. Mr. Benton, in his "Grazier's Ready Reckoner," states that for a half fattened ox, one stone in every twenty must be deducted;

and when they are very fat, one-twentieth may be added. No tables can, however, be at all times implicitly relied upon, as there are many circumstances connected with the build of the animal, the mode of fattening, &c., that will influence the measurement, and consequently the weight. As a general guide, such tables must be useful to the farmer, or grazier, for whose use they are of course principally intended.

TO CURE SHEEP SKINS WITH THE WOOL ON.

Take a spoonful of alum, and two of saltpetre; pulverize and mix well together, then sprinkle the powder on the flesh side of the skin, and lay the two flesh sides together, leaving the wool outside. Then fold up the whole skin as tight as you can and hang in a dry place: in two or three days, as soon as dry, take down, and scrape with a blunt knife till clean and supple; this completes the process, and makes you, a most excellent saddle cover. If, when you kill your mutton, you treat the skins in this way, you can get more for them from the saddlers than you can for the wool and skin separately disposed of otherwise.

N. B. Other skins which you desire to cure with the fur or hair on may be treated in the same way.

S. W. Farmer.

A VALUABLE

COLLECTION OF RECEIPTS

FOR

THE CURE OF DISEASES OF MAN;

AND

FOR OTHER PURPOSES, IN THE MEDICAL DEPARTMENT.

WITH AN INDEX.

RECEIPTS

FOR

THE CURE OF DISEASES OF MAN.

ON BATHING.

If every morning, and, when the heat is oppressive, every evening, the whole surface of the body were bathed in water, fresh from the pump or well, with a sponge or rubbed well with the hands, so that the pores of the skin are rubbed open, and cleansed or rubbed dry with a crash towel (better than a flesh-brush), the population of the city and country in which so excellent a custom prevailed would be remarkable for health, let the climate be as it might. A strong nerve and solidity of flesh would be gained by the process, which would set the heat of summer and the cold of winter at defiance. Thousands of diseases which now haunt our crowded communities would become obsolete. Thirst would not be so much affected, and the temptation to deluge the stomach with fluids would be removed. Perhaps among all the evil practices which produce disease and weakness, none is more injurious, as well as prevalent, than the universal habit of impairing and preventing digestion by filling the stomach with fluids. As we remarked before, a healthy state of the skin would diminish the practice by taking away the inducement. Upon mothers, nurses, and others who have charge of children the frequent lavations of their little charge cannot be too much urged. Physicians tell us that two-thirds of the infantile diseases which occur owe their origin and their aggravation to a neglect of cleanliness. It is not enough that a child's face is not marked with filth so as to be discernible at half a block's distance; the whole body should be so frequently washed that the skin may perform the functions for which nature intended and curiously constructed it.

ANOTHER.—The annexed rules (which experience has established, and physiology approved) are submitted for the benefit of bathers :—1. Bathe one hour before breakfast, or what is much better, one hour before dinner. 2. The stomach should always be empty when we bathe. 3. Never take the cold bath when the temperature of the body is below the natural standard. 4. To prepare the tepid bath, which is the best in a warm climate, the rule should be this : Bring the water to that temperature which feels neither hot nor cold to the arm, or some part of the body usually covered, and after entering the bath raise its heat to that point which imparts the most agreeable feeling. 5. We should take exercise before and after the warm bath; the importance of this is every day evinced where bathing is practised. 6. After leaving the water, the body should be briskly wiped with a coarse towel, and immediately covered with sufficient clothing to excite or preserve the healthy temperature. 7. We should never remain long in the water; from ten to fifteen minutes is sufficient. 8. Every second or third day is often enough to take the bath.

THE TIME REQUIRED TO DIGEST DIFFERENT ARTICLES OF FOOD.

	HOURS	MIN.
Boiled rice	1	00
Sago, tapioca, barley, and boiled milk	2	15
Tripe, and pig's feet	1	00
Fowls, beeves' liver	2	30
Hard eggs	3	30
Soft eggs	3	00
Custard	2	45
Trout, boiled or fried	1	30
Other fresh fish	3	00
Beef rare, roasted	3	00
Dry, roasted	3	30
Salt beef, with mustard	2	30
Pickled pork	4	30
Raw pork	3	00
Roasted pork, fat and lean	5	15
Fried pork	4	15
Stewed pork	3	00
Mutton broiled	3	00
Mutton boiled	3	00
Veal fried	4	30
Fowls boiled	4	00
Fowls roasted	4	00
Ducks roasted	4	00
Wild ducks roasted	4	30
Suet, fresh beef, boiled	5	00
Suet, mutton, boiled	4	30
Butter melted	3	30
Mutton, fresh	3	15
Veal, fresh, broiled	4	00
Wheat bread, fresh baked	3	30
Corn bread	3	15
Sponge cake	2	30
Apple dumplings	3	00
Apples, sweet and mellow	1	30
Apples, sour and mellow	2	00
Parsnips, boiled	2	30
Potatoes, boiled	3	30

Potatoes, roasted	2	30
Raw cabbage	2	30
Raw, with vinegar	2	00
Cabbage, boiled	4	30
Cheese, old	3	30
Soup, beef, vegetables, and bread	4	00
Barley soup	1	30
Chicken soup	3	00
Oyster soup	3	30
Green corn and beans	3	45
Hash, meat and vegetables	2	30
Sausage, fresh broiled	3	20
Codfish, boiled	2	00
Oysters, fresh and raw	2	55
Oysters roasted	3	15
Oysters stewed	3	30
Salmon, salted, boiled	4	00

REMEDY FOR INDIGESTION.

Boil half a pint of white wheat three hours in a quart of water, or a little more if necessary. Drink half a pint of the liquid two or three times a week.

CURE FOR COSTIVENESS.

Take a new-laid egg, raw, add to it three times its bulk of cold water, beat for thirty minutes, take on an empty stomach, and may be taken twice a day; the first time early in the morning, and the second time between eleven and twelve o'clock; increase the quantity to three eggs in the course of ten days. Said to be good for the lungs.

SUPPRESSION OF URINE.

Give about a spoonful of bruised mustard seed in parsley-root tea.

TO PROMOTE URINE.

Beat saffron into powder, mix it up with black soap

and spread it on a piece of leather, and lay it on the navel of the patient; and in one hour's time the effect will appear.

METHOD OF RESTORING LIFE TO THE APPARENTLY DROWNED.

Recommended by the Royal Humane Society of England, instituted in 1774.

Avoid all rough usage. Do not hold up the body by the feet, nor roll it on casks, or rub it with salt, or spirits, or apply tobacco. Lose not a moment in carrying the body to the nearest house, with the hands and shoulders raised. Place it in a warm room, if the weather is cold. Preserve silence, and positively admit no more than three intelligent persons. Let the body be instantly stripped, dried, and wrapped in hot blankets, which are frequently to be renewed. Keep the mouth, nostrils and throat, free and clean. Apply warm substances to the back, spine, pit of the stomach, armpit, and soles of the feet. Rub the body with heated flannels, or cotton, or warm hands. Attempt to restore breathing by gently blowing with a bellows in one nostril, closing the mouth and other nostril. Press down the breast carefully with both hands, and then let it rise again, and thus imitate natural breathing. Keep up the application of heat; continue the rubbing; increase it when life appears, and then give a tea-spoonful of warm water, or very weak brandy and water, or wine and water. Persevere for six hours. Send quickly for medical assistance.

ANIMAL LIFE.

A hare will live ten years; a cat, ten; a goat, eight; an ox, twenty; a hog, twenty-five; a pigeon, eight; a turtle dove, twenty-five; a raven, one hundred; an eagle, one hundred; and a goose, one hundred and fifty.

GESTATION.

The period of gestation, or the length of time which different animals go with young, should be known by every farmer; that the season of copulation with his different kinds of stock may be so regulated as to have them bring forth their young under the most favourable circumstances.

Mares go a few days over eleven months with foal. Cows go about forty weeks, or ten lunar months. Ewes bring forth at the end of five months. Goats, at four-and-a-half months. Sows, at four months.

The term of incubation, or time which different fowls sit upon their eggs before hatching, is as follows:—

Swans sit six weeks; turkeys sit thirty days; geese from twenty-seven to thirty days; ducks, from twenty-seven to thirty days; hens, twenty-one days; pigeons, or doves, fifteen days.

REMEDY IN CASE OF SWALLOWING PINS, FISH, OR OTHER SHARP BONES.

Administer four grains of tartar emetic in warm water, and let the patient drink the white from six eggs, which, coagulating upon the stomach before the tartar operates, envelopes the piece or bone, and it is brought up. A person who had swallowed several pins was made to throw up the whole by the above method.

TO CLEANSE THE TEETH, AND IMPROVE THE BREATH.

To four ounces of fresh prepared lime water add one drachm of Peruvian bark, and wash the teeth with the water in the morning before breakfast, and after supper. It will effectually destroy the tartar on the teeth, and remove the offensive smell arising from those decayed.

TO STOP BLOOD.

It has been found that soot applied to a fresh wound will not only stop the bleeding, but ease the pain.

N. Y. Farmer.

BLEEDING AT THE NOSE.

Bathe in vinegar.

TO STOP VOMITING.

Give parsley tea, of the roots and tops.

FROST BITTEN.

Bathe in warm beef pickle.

BURDON'S EXCELLENT OINTMENT.

Yellow resin, the size of a hen's egg, to be melted in an earthen pot over a slow fire, to which add the same quantity of beeswax; when melted add half a pound of hog's lard, and, when that is dissolved, add two ounces of honey, and half a pound of common turpentine, and keep gently boiling a few minutes, stirring all the time; take it off the fire, and when it has cooled a little, stir into it two ounces of verdigris, finely powdered; then give the whole a few minutes gentle boiling, and pour through a sieve for use. Nothing takes fire out of a burn or scald in human flesh so soon as this ointment. I would suggest that no store in a newly settled district ought to be without a plentiful supply of the above ointment for sale. It is equally good for cuts and bruises and putrefying sores, and might be denominated, with propriety, the universal remedy.   JAMES PEDDER.

TO MAKE OPODELDOC.

Take of Castile soap, powdered, three ounces; camphor, one ounce; brandy, one pint. Dissolve the soap in the spirits, by the fire, then add the camphor.

POWDER OF SLIPPERY ELM.

We live but to learn and obtain knowledge. Being in the country a few days since, on a visit to a sick friend, I was shown an article entirely new to me, which is said to be remarkably nutritious and palatable for debilitated and sick persons. It was flour prepared by the Shakers from slippery elm, and used the same as arrowroot. One tablespoonful of this flour, boiled in a pint of new milk, is excellent to feed infants weaned from the breast. They will not only fatten upon it, but it will prevent bowel complaints. It makes an easy and nutritious diet for consumptive and dyspeptic persons. From the character I received of it, I presume that it only need be known to become of general use.—*United States Gazette.*

CURE FOR THE BITE OF THE VIPER, RATTLESNAKE.

In great cities, particularly in London, a number of persons procure their livelihood by catching vipers. They are employed by chemists, apothecaries, &c. I remember some years before leaving England, to have read in the Royal Society, in London, a curious circumstance of one of these viper-catchers. A member of the society had casually received information that a man engaged in this business was frequently bitten, and that he cured himself with sweet oil. After considerable inquiry, the viper-catcher was found, and the questions asked whether he cured himself by the oil, and whether he was willing to satisfy a number of gentlemen of the fact. The man answered in the affirmative to both questions. Accordingly a very numerous meeting of the Royal Society was convened, composed of a considerable number of nobility. The viper-catcher attended, accompanied by his wife and a large viper; and laying his arm naked to the shoulder, suffered the irritated reptile to strike, which it did very forcibly. His wife permitted the poison to operate till her husband's head, face and tongue, were greatly swollen, his arm and face turned very black, and his senses much affected, when she applied the oil by pouring a small quantity down him, and bathing the part bitten. The man gradually recovered. The circumstance being strongly impressed upon my mind, and knowing the poison of an English viper is considered in that country the most venomous in nature, determined me to try its power in the bite of a rattlesnake the first opportunity that should offer in the district that I reside in. In 1766 I was travelling through Pendleton, S. C., and met a man who inquired of me if I could assist to relieve the pain of a person who had been bitten by a large rattlesnake. Although sorry for the man's misfortune, I rejoiced at the opportunity I had offered to ascertain fully the properties of sweet oil as an antidote to this deadly poison. Having a phial of this oil in my pocket, I hastened to the suffering creature, and on seeing him, his appearance struck me as the most frightful I had ever beheld. His head and face were extremely swollen, and the latter black; his tongue proportionably enlarged, and extending out of his mouth; his eyes appeared as if they would shoot from their sockets, and his senses gave every appearance of death. He had been bitten on the side of the foot. I immediately, but with great difficulty, poured down him two tablespoonsful of the oil. Its effects were almost instantaneous, and exceedingly powerful in counteracting the poison, as appeared by the strong though quick convulsions which followed. In about thirty minutes it operated strongly, both as an emetic and cathartic, after which the swelling of the head, face, &c., gradually abated, and the tongue began to assume its place. In two hours he was so far recovered as to articulate, and from that time recovered fast till he got perfectly over it. The oil inwardly taken, and externally applied, did not exceed seven spoonsful. The number of cases of the like nature in twelve years has been considerable to which sweet oil has proved itself to be peculiarly adapted, and fully adequate to the worst of cases, if timely applied. It is a remedy which every person can command (when others cannot be procured), and ought not to be without. Indeed, many cautious persons have carried a small phial of oil constantly about them. It has also been used with equal success when horses, cattle, dogs, &c., have been bitten. One case I am credibly informed, occurred where the oil succeeded when given to a woman who had been bitten by a small dog, and who exhibited strong symptoms of hydrophobia. I can hardly excuse myself of criminal neglect in having so long omitted to make thus public this sovereign remedy for the worst of poisons. The knowledge of the efficacy of the sweet oils abundantly diffused in the district of Pendleton, and partially so in some of the adjoining districts, and wishing it to be known generally, caused me to write these remarks for publication.—*Augusta Constitutionalist.*

ANOTHER.—A weed with a smooth leaf, and bulbous, milky root, known by the name of "Lion's tongue," when applied in a proper manner, I have never known fail. Manner of application: take a handful of the roots, wash clean, and boil in sweet milk. Let the patient drink occasionally of the milk thus boiled, and apply the root as a poultice o the wound, keeping it moist with the milk.—*Gen. Farm.*

ANOTHER.—The most simple and convenien t reme dy I have ever heard of is alum. A piece the size of a hickory nut, dissolved in water and drank, or chewed and swallowed, is sufficient. I have good authority for saying that it has been tried many times on men and dogs, and that they have invariably recovered. I know of some planters whose hands are exposed to be bitten by rattlesnakes, who keep themselves always provided with it in their pockets, and that they have several times found use for it.
Macon Messenger.

ONIONS AN ANTIDOTE FOR POISON.

Upward of forty years ago I knew a man who wilfully took eleven grains of arsenic in warm tea, in order to kill himself. I took immediately three physicians, who exerted their skill to save him; but to no purpose; he said he must die. By their consent another person proposed onions, which were immediately applied to his stomach, arm-pits, wrists, and all the tender parts of his body. Though he was much swelled, he immediately began to recover, and the next day went to his work. It appeared like a miracle to all who witnessed it.

CURE FOR HYDROPHOBIA.

Take two ounces of the fresh leaves of the treebox; two ounces of the fresh leaves of rue; one half ounce of sage; chop these fine, and boil in a pint of water, down to a half pint; strain carefully, and press out the liquor very firmly. Put back the ingredients again, and add a pint of milk, and boil down again to half a pint, and strain as before; then mix both liquors together, of which give one-third part each subsequent morning, fasting. As it possesses no power to relieve the disease itself, but is given merely as a preventive, any time between the reception of the bite and the first appearance of the symptoms is the proper period for administering it.

ANOTHER.—For the bite of a mad dog, let the person bit, immediately drink a pint of good white wine vinegar; repeat this three mornings fasting, and wash the part well with vinegar at the fire; then take a large spoonful of the juice of rue three mornings fasting; after the vinegar, before you take the rue, let about eight ounces of blood be taken away.

ANTIDOTE FOR POISON BY ARSENIC.

Salad or olive oil taken warm, and repeated occasionally, will infallibly prevent any bad consequences, if the arsenic has not been taken very long before. It is the true antidote for arsenic, and should immediately be made use of, as soon as it is discovered that any person has swallowed it by mistake or otherwise. A gentle vomit given just after taking it, and then repeatedly drinking very fat mutton broth, will effectually cure it; by this method, Sir Hans Sloane saved the life of a young man, who, at his house at Chelsea, had drank a quantity of milk, into which arsenic had been put to poison rats.

CURE FOR CHOLERA MORBUS.

The worst cases of cholera morbus, dysentery, bloody flux, &c., that I ever saw, I have repeatedly cured in a few minutes or hours, by a strong tea made of the bark of the sweet-gum; taken green from the tree is best; steep a handful in a pint of water, until the liquor is like good coffee; drink it clear, or sweetened with loaf sugar, or add a glass of good French brandy, if the attack is very severe.   S. ROBINSON.

We can add our testimony to the nature of the sweet-gum tea; having experienced amazing and speedy relief from its use, in a violent case of dysentery, which refused to yield to the usual remedies.

We have also seen, in the last five years, its wonderful benefits in many other cases. We have used the decoction made from the bark, both green and dried, and have discovered no material difference in the effect, both being efficacious.—*Franklin Farmer*.

CURE FOR GANGRENE.

In an account of a fight between a party of Waccos Tawachanies Indians, and a small party of Americans, in Texas, in November, 1831, recently published in the Philadelphia Post, we find the following singular method of curing the leg of one of the party, which was shattered during the action, by a musket ball. It was lucky for David Buchannan that no surgeon attended the party, or he would have been a leg shorter all his days.

David Buchannan's wounded leg here mortified; and having no surgical instruments, nor medicine of any kind, not even a dose of salts, we boiled some live oak bark very strong, and thickened it with powdered charcoal and Indian meal; made a poultice of it, and tied it round his leg, over which we sewed a Buffalo skin, and travelled along five days without looking at it. When it was opened, the mortified parts had all dropped off, and it was in a fair way for healing, which it finally did, and is as well now as ever it was.

CURE, OR PREVENTION OF SPASMS.

Mr. Miller—I beg leave to inform the public,

through you, that in a home practice of thirty years, I have lost but one patient by spasms, and that was the first case I ever saw. The cure is simple and within the reach of any one. It is as follows: lacerate, or scarify the part punctured, stung, or bitten, whether by splinter, nail, spider, or snake, so as to cause blood to flow; and into the part wounded rub saltpetre, very finely powdered. It is instantaneous in its effects. One quarter of an hour will give relief to pain passing through the system. If it be any length of time after the accident before the means of relief by the nitre be applied, it will be well to envelope the limb in woollen, and bathe in strong warm ley; and to give internally spirits of turpentine, or hartshorn and olive, lamp, or sweet oil.—*James King, Sen., Pon Pon, September,* 1836.

TO CURE SALT RHEUM.

Take one quart of tar; add two gallons of water; let it stand two or three days, stirring it occasionally. Then soak or pour off the water, and put into bottles. Take half a teacupful three times a day before eating. The following ointment should be made and used externally, while drinking tar water: take the yolk of an egg; the same size of fresh butter; half the size of tar; one teaspoonful pulverized cream of tartar. Mix them together with the point of a knife, until it becomes a perfect salve; anoint the parts affected three times a day with this ointment, and the cure is effected in two weeks. General Richard Shaw, of Newport, Rhode Island, says he has by this remedy cured a number of persons of this fretting disease in two weeks, and has never known a failure, where the remedy was applied according to the directions.—[Communicated by S. H. Weed.]—*Portsmouth Jour.*

CURE FOR THE STING OF A WASP OR BEE.

Apply an onion, by binding it to the part affected, which is stated to be a certain cure.

ANOTHER.—Bind on the place a thick plaster of common salt moistened; it will soon extract the venom.

CURE FOR A CANCER WART.

Apply a plaster of tar and mutton suet, and drink plentifully of tar water, made pretty strong.

CURE FOR THE CANCER.

Mr. Thomas Tyrrell, of Missouri, advertises that a cancer upon his nose, which had been treated without success by Dr. Smith of Newhaven, and the ablest surgeons in the western country, has been cured in the following manner:—He was recommended to use a strong potash, made of the ley of ashes of red oak bark, boiled down to the consistence of molasses, to cover the cancer with, and in about an hour afterward cover this with a plaster of tar, which must be removed after a few days, and if any protuberances remain in the wound, apply more potash to them, and the plaster again, until they all disappear; after which heal the wound with any common salve. Dentery and the knife had been used in vain. This treatment effected a speedy and perfect cure.

ANOTHER.—Take of red clover blossoms four pounds, roots and tops of narrow dock, one pound; boil in water till the strength is out, then drain and put the juice back into the kettle and boil, taking care not to burn it, until reduced to the consistence of salve.

CURE FOR A WEN.

Make a very strong brine, and dip in it a piece of flannel two or three times doubled, and apply it to the wen, keeping it constantly wet night and day until a separation takes place.

CURE FOR TETTER OR RINGWORM.

After I had the tetter-worm for nearly twenty years on my hand, and had used dollars' worth of celebrated tetter ointment, which took off the skin repeatedly, without effecting a cure, a friend advised me to take some blood-root (called also red-root, Indian paint, &c.), slice it in vinegar, and afterwards wash the place affected, with the liquid. I suppose the vinegar extracted the strength out of the root, for in a few days the dry scurf was removed, and my diseased hand appeared as whole as the other. I could scarcely believe that a perfect cure was so speedily accomplished by this simple remedy; but as nearly two years have passed without the least appearance of its return, I need no longer doubt the fact, and for the benefit of others I wish the value of the red-root more generally known.

The red-root grows about a foot high in rich woodland, and flowers in April. The leaf is roundish and deeply indented, somewhat like the white-oak leaves, stems naked, supporting single flowers, blossoms white. When the fresh root, which is about the size of the little finger, and blood red, is broken, a juice issues in large drops resembling blood.

CURE FOR A FELON.

Bathe the part affected in ashes and water; take the yolk of an egg, six drops of spirits of turpentine, a few beet-leaves cut fine, a small quantity of hard soap, one teaspoonful of snuff, or fine tobacco; then add one tablespoonful of burned salt, and one of Indian meal, and it never fails to effect a cure. To be applied as a poultice.

ANOTHER.—Take of rock or of any other table salt,

one ounce, hard soap one ounce, spirits of turpentine half an ounce, roast the salt, rolled in a cabbage leaf or wet paper, for twenty or thirty minutes, then pulverize it, mix with the soap previously shaved down, and add the spirits of turpentine, which will make a soft salve or poultice. This must be applied to the affected part, and renewed as often as it becomes dry. If applied before matter is formed, it will prevent its formation by three or four hours' application : if not applied until matter is formed, it will stop its progress, but the matter must be let out, when the ulcer will be healed by the same means as in any other case of the like kind.

CURE FOR THE ITCH.

Take black pepper, ginger, and brimstone, each of equal parts, a little West India rum, and a little lard; all well mixed as salve. Rub a little in your hands, hold them to the fire, and smell for à few minutes; repeat it several times in the day and night.

CURE FOR THE POLYPUS IN THE NOSE.

In conversation with a friend from the western country, I have been informed of a fact, too important, as it appears to me, to be withheld from the public. His daughter was troubled with a polypus in the nose, which was extracted by a surgeon, but soon grew again to its former size. He heard of the blood-root as a cure, and it was tried with such efficacy that the polypus shrivelled away in ten days, and was soon entirely gone.

Another young woman in the same neighbourhood had one so large as to spread her nostrils considerably, and affect her speech. After using the blood-root a short time, the polypus dropped out entire, and she was soon well.

Receipt.—Take one half ounce of blood-root finely pulverized, and sift it, and one drachm of calomel; mix them together for a sternutatory. A small pinch of this powder is to be snuffed up the nostril three times a day, and a syringe of the following wash is to be thrown up the nostril twice a day:—Dissolve half an ounce of powdered alum in a gill of brandy; shake the phial until it is dissolved.

ANOTHER.—Take of blood-root and bayberry-root bark equal parts mixed, made fine, and used as a snuff several times a day.

CURE FOR THE DROPSY.

Take cinders from a blacksmith's shop, and beat them fine, sift them, take out the coarse particles; mix the fine cinders with a pint of honey until it is stiff enough to lie on the point of a case knife, not hard like pills. Give the patient as much as will lie on the point of a case-knife three times a day, morning, noon, and night. This mixture is very purgative, and will cause the patient to discharge great quantities of water, both purgatively and by urine. The potion may be given according to the operation: if the quantity appears to be too severe, give less; if it does not operate enough, give more, and continue it until the swelling is gone.

The patient may eat any diet but milk, of which he should not taste a drop; neither use any other medicine while taking the above. I have known several persons cured of that dreadful disease by using the above mixture; some were so bad that the water oozed out of their feet and legs, and left their tracks as they walked on the floor.

Another.—Water, two quarts; whiskey, one quart; ground ginger, two tablespoonsful ; Peruvian bark, two spoonsful ; copperas, two spoonsful; all well mixed together. Dose, one or two tablespoonsful, night and morning ; drink freely of ginger tea through the day; abstain from milk, and all kinds of grease, while using the medicine. Shake the bottle well when a dose is to be taken.

Another.—A correspondent informs us that there is a boy living at Deumy, who about three months ago was seized with dropsy, for which he underwent the operation of tapping ; after which the water again gathering, the boy was so much swelled that the two doctors who attended him said he must be tapped a second time, in a day or two. It happened, however, that a boy went to see the one affected with the dropsy, who mentioned to the other that he had a strong desire to eat some onions. The boy went home to his father's house and procured some for him, and what is remarkable, in a short time after eating them the swelling abated, the boy discharged a great quantity of water, and continues to do so : he eats onions every day, and is now walking about. Raw onions in this case seem to have produced an astonishing result, which for the benefit of persons similarly afflicted ought to be known.—*Glasgow Chronicle.*

CURE FOR THE GRAVEL.

The excruciating sufferings sustained by persons afflicted by gravel in the kidneys, &c., induced me to communicate a remedy which has in many instances afforded relief. This remedy was discovered and its efficacy first tested by Dr. Williams, a late eminent physician in Virginia. He had for several years suffered extremely by gravel. As an experiment, Dr. Williams put a small quantity of the gravel which he had voided into three wine glasses, one containing gin, a second containing a solution of lime (lime water), the third glass containing pure strong coffee. After waiting a few days, on examination, he found that the gravel deposited in gin was not in the slightest degree altered; that in lime water appeared a little softened; that deposited in strong coffee was reduced to an impalpable powder.

Encouraged by this experiment, Dr. Williams immediately adopted the use of pure strong coffee, not mixed with sugar, milk, or any ingredient. In a short time he voided gravel, reduced to sand, with little pain, and was relieved. The above important facts were stated to me by a respectable physician, who has administered the remedy with similar success.

J. M.

ANOTHER.—Make a strong tea of blackberry brier root; add some Virginia snake root; while this is steeping, give the patient freely of cayenne or composition powders; then drink freely of the tea, and in fifteen minutes after drinking this tea, give two teaspoonsful of the pulverized butterfly or pleurisy root in a teacupful of hot water sweetened; repeat both every half hour alternately for ten or twelve hours; then use a tea of parsley three or four days.

CURE FOR THE PILES.

A cure for this most painful disorder has always been considered by those afflicted with it of the first importance. The writer of this has, for the last five years, suffered under that inveterate disease, during which time he could obtain no relief, until he accidentally met with a person who gave him a receipt which effected in him a complete cure, and he now, from motives of humanity, makes it known to the public, viz.:—Take a lump of strong British alum, about two inches in length, which smoothe down with a knife to the thickness of three quarters of an inch; apply this morning and evening, first wetting it in cold water. In five to seven days the cure will be complete.—*New York paper.*

CURE FOR THE DYSENTERY.

Take a teaspoonful of the compound syrup of rhubarb, and a teaspoonful of paregoric, in a little sweetened water, three times a day if necessary—to be continued until a cure is effected.

For children; mix a full dose for a grown person, and give it in broken doses, according to age.

ANOTHER, FOR DYSENTERY.—Take of the bark of the roots of wild cherry tree, and poplar bark, equal parts, and make a strong tea by moderate steeping, strain off and add to each gallon four pounds of loaf sugar, four ounces of the finely pulverized kernels of peach stones, and two quarts of good French brandy. Dose, half a wine glass full several times a day.

CURE FOR THE CROUP.

Cut onions into thin slices; between and over them put brown sugar; when the sugar is dissolved, a teaspoonful of the syrup will produce almost instantaneous relief. This simple and effectual remedy for this distressing malady should be known to all persons having the care of children.

Cause of croup in infants.—Eberle, in his excellent work on the diseases of children, says that the mode of dressing infants with their necks and upper part of the breast bare, cannot fail to render them subject to the influence of cold, and its dangerous consequences. In the country, especially among the Germans, who are in the habit of clothing their children in such a manner as to leave no part of the breast and lower portion of the neck exposed, croup is an exceeding rare disease. Whereas in cities, or among people who adopt the modes of dress common in cities, this frightful disease is in proportion to the population vastly more frequent.

ANOTHER.—If a child is taken with the croup, instantly apply cold water, ice water if possible, suddenly and freely to the neck and chest with a sponge —the breathing will almost instantly be relieved; so soon as possible let the sufferer drink as much as it can, then wipe it dry, cover it up warm, and soon a quiet slumber will relieve the parent's anxiety.

CURE FOR WORMS IN CHILDREN.

A writer in the Farmer's Register, who, being a slaveholder, has a large family under his care, says that for nearly thirty years he has found the following preparation a certain cure for worms: " Take the fat of old bacon, sliced, and fried in a pan until the essence is all out of it, take out the rind first, then put in as much wormseed (vulgarly called Jerusalem oak) as is necessary, as much sugar or molasses as will make it palatable, and give it three mornings in succession. The children will eat it freely—some you will have to restrain from eating too much. Incredible as it may appear, I have known as many as one hundred and twenty or thirty large worms come from a child three or four years old. I usually give the medicine spring and fall.

Another for Worms.—Butternut syrup, one tablespoonful; composition two tablespoonsful; castor oil one tablespoonful. Give in small doses until relief is obtained.

A REMEDY FOR ARSENIC.

Tobacco is said to be an infallible preventative against the fatal effects of arsenic, when taken into the stomach. In several instances where tobacco juice was swallowed after taking arsenic, no sickness resulted from the use of the tobacco and not the least harm from the arsenic. This is an important discovery.

A CURE FOR CORNS.

Dip a small piece of cotton in lamp or whale oil, apply it to the corn, and wrap a bandage round it; repeat this for six or eight days, and the corn becomes soft, and is easily removed. The experiment has been tried with success.

A CURE FOR THRUSH.

The root called Hog's Tush may be mashed fine, and steeped in a little water for two or three hours, then the mouth may be washed with the liquor sweetened with sugar, two or three times in the course of a day. This is a never failing remedy, and generally two or three applications are sufficient.

CURE FOR SUMMER COMPLAINTS.

We are indebted to a friend for the following receipt for making blackberry syrup, said to be almost a certain specific for the summer complaint. In 1832 it was successfully used in case of cholera. To two quarts of blackberry juice, add one pound of loaf sugar, half an ounce of allspice. Boil all together for a short time, and when cold add a pint of fourth-proof French brandy. From a teaspoonful to a wine glass may be given at a time, till relieved, according to the age of the patient.

CRAMP IN THE STOMACH.

Take a pint of warm water, sweeten it well with molasses, and put in a teaspoonful of Cayenne, and drink freely of it; at the same time heat the feet well by the fire, or put them into warm water, which will afford speedy relief.

ANOTHER.—Drink plentifully of a strong tea made of the blue cohosh root.

CURE FOR WARTS.

These troublesome and often painful excrescences, covering the hands sometimes to the number of a hundred or more, may be destroyed by a simple, safe, and certain application. The writer discovered it accidentally, while performing some chemical experiments with soda. The matter is merely to dissolve as much common washing soda as the water will take up—then wash the hands or warts with this for a minute or two, and allowing them to dry without being wiped. This being repeated two or three days, will gradually destroy the most irritable wart. Its theory appears to be that of warts having a lower power of vitality than the skin, so that the alkali is sufficient to produce the disorganization of the former without affecting the latter. The warts never return.

Phil. Chron.

CURE FOR DEAFNESS.

It is said that by melting sulphuric æther and ammonia, and allowing it to stand fourteen days, a solution is formed, which if properly applied to the internal ear, will remove, in almost every case, this hitherto considered incurable affection.

ANOTHER.—Equal parts of the juice of houseleek, brandy, and sweet oil, in a phial, to be hung up exposed to the sun for a month or more. This dropped in the ear at night, and on wool to be kept in the ear, is a sure remedy for deafness.

ANOTHER.—Syringe the ears well with some warm milk and oil, then take a quarter of an ounce of liquid opodeldoc, and as much oil of almonds; mix them well, and drop a few drops into each ear, stopping them with a little cotton or wool: repeat this every night when going to bed.—*Dr. Feathergill.*

CURE FOR THE GOUT.

The best cure for the gout is to apply a leek poultice to the part affected; numerous instances of its efficacy in this painful disorder have recently occurred. Its culture should be cherished as a medicine of inestimable value.

CURE FOR RHEUMATISM.

BRUNSWICK C. H. Va., Jan. 24, 1835.

To the Editor of the American Farmer.—I have been afflicted with rheumatism three times in my life: the first time, in April, 1822; the second, about one year ago; and the last a few days ago. The first two attacks were not very severe, but continued from two to four weeks. The last was much the most painful and violent. I had been in the habit of using common remedies until lately, several of my neighbours having tried the one I shall now describe. I also resorted to it, and I was entirely relieved in forty-eight hours; and I have never known or heard of a case in which it has not given immediate relief. That no mistake may occur, and that some of your botanical friends may do the plant justice, I herewith inclose you one. It is found in most woodland in this and the adjoining counties; indeed, I have never seen any destitute of it where I have examined; of the limits of the region in which it grows I am ignorant. It is here called wild arsenic, or wild ratsbane, and the most poisonous qualities are ascribed to it. But I had it rubbed on the parts affected, using no extraordinary caution, and nothing has occurred to prove its poisonous properties.

The way to prepare it for use is, to pull it up, wash the dirt off, and put it in a vessel, roots and all, with common whiskey, in such quantity as that after it has steeped for twenty-four hours the liquor assumes a blackish appearance. In this state it is rubbed by some strong hand, on the parts diseased, as hard as the pain will allow, for about fifteen minutes; and also have flannel cloths dipped into it, and spread over the seat of the pain. This is to be repeated three times a day. When I had the flannel cloth applied, the pain was so much increased by it that I was obliged to have it removed in the course of ten or fifteen minutes. In making this communication, sir, I may be doing an act of supererogation, as the remedy is much more extensively known than I had supposed; but if I shall give relief to one individual afflicted with that excruciating malady, I shall feel satisfied for the trouble I have taken, and hope you will excuse that I may have given you. This preparation will lose nothing by age. E. B. HICKS.

STRENGTHENING PLASTER.

Take of resin, beeswax, white turpentine, one pound each; one tablespoonful of black pepper pulverized; one pint of French brandy. Put the whole into a new earthen crock; melt and simmer till the brandy is all evaporated.

ANOTHER may be made by melting turpentine with a sufficient quantity of resin to give it a proper consistence.

CURE FOR WOMEN'S BREASTS SWELLED OR INFLAMED.

Take soft soap, and make strong suds, and with a flannel cloth saturated with the suds wash and rub the breast downward with some degree of violence, once an hour, after which each time bathe the breast with polecat oil, or some soft grease and camphor. Keep the breast close covered with flannel.

ANOTHER.—Take hard soap and common salt, each two ounces, new milk half a pint; shave the soap fine; put all into a vessel, and simmer slowly over a fire. Take care not to burn. When hot, stir in a spoonful of corn meal. Spread all on one cloth, and cover the whole breasts. The surface of the poultice should be covered with soft grease, and the plaster should be applied as hot as can be borne. A new poultice to be applied every three hours till relief is given.

REMEDY FOR BURNS.

Dear Sir,—I have so often seen remedies for human ills given to the newspapers, and at once consigned to oblivion, that I have for a great while hesitated to present this remedy to the public. For fourteen years I have prescribed it and witnessed its healing effect. I deliberately say, from fourteen years' experience, that no disease or injury to the human system has a more certain remedy than this for the most distressing of all injuries, that of scalds and burns. The relief is almost instantaneous: for a minute to half an hour will usually find a full relief from pain, no matter what the extent of the burn, even if the skin is removed from the body. The first knowledge I had of it was the almost miraculous cure of a little boy who fell into a half-hogshead of boiling water, prepared for scalding hogs. The entire person and limbs of the boy passed under the scalding water up to the chin, so as to scald his whole neck. On removing his clothes, nearly all the skin followed from his neck, hands, arms, chest, back, abdomen, and almost every bit of skin from his lower extremities. In this deplorable condition, literally flayed alive with scalding water, the remedy was applied, as a momentary application, until the physicians should arrive. Two eminent physicians soon came, and on hearing of the extent of the scald, pronounced it a certainly fatal case, and directed the boy to remain with the remedy over him until he should die. In six weeks he was restored quite well, with scarcely a scar on his person or limbs. The remedy increases in value from the fact, that, under almost all circumstances, it may be obtained. It is as follows:—Take soot from a chimney where wood is burned, rub it fine, and mix one part of soot with three parts or nearly so of hogs' lard, fresh butter, or any kind of fresh grease that is not salted. Spread this on linen, or muslin, or any cotton, for easier or more perfect adaptation. If in very extensive burns or scalds, the cloth should be torn into strips before putting over the scald: let the remedy be freely and fully applied, so as perfectly to cover all the burned parts. No other application is required until the patient is well, except to apply fresh applications of the soot and lard. In steamboat explosions this remedy can in nearly all cases be at once applied; and if done, many valuable lives would be saved, and a vast amount of suffering alleviated.

A Physician of Philadelphia.

RINGWORM.

Take of the juice from the hull around the black walnuts, after they have got their growth; and rub it well on the ringworm. Three or four daily applications will be sufficient.

DR. BLAKE'S REMEDY FOR TOOTHACHE.

A remedy for this most painful affliction, which has succeeded in ninety-five cases out of a hundred, is alum reduced to an impalpable powder two drachms, nitrous spirits of æther, seven drachms, mixed and applied to the tooth.

ANOTHER.—Make a solution of camphor and pulverised Cayenne pepper: dip this in a small quantity of raw cotton, and apply it to the affected tooth, and it will give instant relief. To prevent the composition from getting to the throat, lay a bit of rag over it for a few moments.

A CURE FOR THE EAR-ACHE.

Take a large onion, bore a hole two-thirds through, large enough to contain a tablespoonful of sweet oil; roast and press out the juice, add a little laudanum, wet a little cotton with the liquid, and put it in the ear.

EYE-WATER, FOR CURE OF SORE EYES.

Take white vitriol, a lump about the size of a pea, and a lump twice that size of loaf sugar, three cloves pulverized, and well mixed, a hen's egg, roasted or boiled very hard; peel off the shell, cut through the middle, and take out the yolk; put the aforesaid powder into the hollow where the yolk was; place the two halves of the egg together again, wrap it in a strong cloth, and wring it hard; do not have too much cloth around the egg; wring quickly; drop one drop of the juice in the eye, or dip the finger in the liquid, and touch the corner of the eye at pleasure.

ANOTHER—FOR CHRONIC SORE EYES.

One ounce lobelia seed, one ounce Cayenne pepper seed, one ounce gum myrrh, one ounce lady's slipper, half an ounce camphor, and of alcohol one pint; pulverize and mix them together, set it in the sun ten days, shake it often, and strain it in a bottle for use.

REMEDY FOR FILMS ON THE EYE.

A correspondent of the New England Farmer gives the following recipe for removing films from the eyes of animals, of the efficacy of which we have no doubt. Several years since a son of ours had films formed on his eyes, which we removed by dropping a small portion of molasses on his eye-lids when asleep, for three or four nights in succession. He was so restless, and resisted the application so resolutely when awake, that we had to avail ourselves of the opportunity afforded by his slumbers to apply the remedy:

Directions for using.—Mix one teaspoonful of the drops with three of new milk, and apply it to the eyes for three days: then mix one teaspoonful of the drops with two of new milk, and apply this three days; then mix equal quantities of the drops and milk, and apply till cured.

"Perhaps all your readers do not know the easiest, as well as most effectual remedy for removing a film from the eye of an animal. It is simply to put a teaspoonful of molasses on the eye-ball. I have relieved oxen, horses, cows and sheep in this manner, and know of no other equal to it."

Glenburn, Maine, Dec. 5th, 1843.

REMEDY FOR COLDS.

The following receipt to cure a cold is said to be so efficacious that we republish it at the request of a correspondent, who has tested its virtues. Take a large teaspoonful of flaxseed, with half a stick of liquorice, and a quarter of a pound of raisins; put them into two quarts of soft water, and let it simmer over a slow fire till it is reduced to one; then add to it a quarter of a pound of brown sugar candy pounded, a tablespoonful of white wine vinegar, or lemon juice.

NOTE.—The vinegar is best to be added only to that quantity you are going to take, for if it be put into the whole, it is liable in a little time to grow flat. Drink half a pint at going to bed, and take a little when the cough is troublesome.

The receipt generally cures the worst colds in two or three days; and if taken in time may be said to be an almost infallible remedy. It is a sovereign balsam cordial for the lungs, without the opening qualities which endanger fresh colds on going out. It has been known to cure colds that have almost been settled into consumptions in less than three weeks.

TO CURE A COUGH, OR COLD.

The editor of the Baltimore Farmer and Gardener says, that the best remedy he ever tried in his family for a cough, or cold, is a decoction of the leaves of the pine tree, sweetened with loaf sugar, to be freely drank warm, when going to bed at night, and cold through the day.

CURE FOR A COUGH.

Take equal parts of the moss that grows on white oak, white maple, and white ash trees; mix, and make a strong tea; sweeten, and drink freely.

CURE FOR A WHOOPING-COUGH.

Take equal parts of sweet oil, honey, and vinegar, and simmer together over a fire. Dose, a teaspoonful, or more, if necessary.

Another.—Take a good handful of dried colt's foot leaves, cut them small and boil them in a pint of water, till half a pint is boiled away; then take it off the fire, and when it is almost cold, strain it through a cloth, squeezing the herb as dry as you can; and then throw it away, and dissolve in the liquor an ounce of sugar candy, finely powdered; and then give the child (if it be about three or four years old, and so in proportion) one spoonful of it, cold or warm as the seasons prove, three or four times a day, or oftener if the fits of coughing come frequently, till well, which will be in a few days.

CURE FOR THE ASTHMA.

One ounce pulverized columbo, one ounce lobelia herb, one ounce hira picra, one ounce skunk cabbage, one ounce asafœtida, one ounce ginger, one ounce elecampane, one ounce nerve powder, one ounce rhubarb, one ounce hoarhound, and two quarts good gin. One wine-glassful twice a day.

CURE FOR INFLUENZA.

Take equal parts of good vinegar and water: to a teacupful of this mixture add one spoonful of Cayenne; sweeten with honey or sugar. Dose, a tablespoonful at going to bed, and one during the night, if the cough be troublesome.

ANOTHER.—Cover four or five eggs with vinegar or lime juice, and let them remain until the shells are dissolved, then mix with them honey, candy, and sweet oil, of each half a pint. Take a tablespoonful every three or four hours.

CURE FOR SORE THROAT.

Take a small piece of alum in your mouth, and let it dissolve, spitting out your spittle till it is all dissolved, a little before going to bed, without rinsing your mouth.

PUTRID SORE THROAT.

Take one ounce of Jesuit's bark, one ounce of gum myrrh, boil both in two quarts of water over a gentle fire; strain it, and give a tablespoonful every hour, after gargling with sage, honey, and saltpetre.

CURE FOR CHOLIC.

One ounce of cloves, two ounces of cinnamon, two ounces of ginger root pared, two ounces of allspice, three drachms oil of lavender, one and a half pints of alchohol; pulverize and mix together. Set it in the sun for ten days, shake often, then strain, and it will be fit for use. Dose, a teaspoonful on sugar, according to circumstances, till relief is obtained.

CURE FOR HEARTBURN.

A teacupful of camomile tea, or a small quantity of chalk, scraped into a glass of water: or a small teaspoonful of magnesia in a glass of water.

CURE FOR JAUNDICE.

Take of the bark of the wild cherry-tree, and the bark of sassafras root, which steep in good rum, and take a glass in the morning.

CURE FOR PALSY.

Perpetual blisters are serviceable, and the following drops have frequently afforded great benefit; take sal volatile drops half an ounce, lavender drops and tincture of castor, a quarter of an ounce; mix them together. Dose, is forty drops frequently in a glass of wine and water: or half a drachm of wild valerian root in powder may be taken three times a day. The diet should be warm and attenuating.

CURE FOR MEASLES.

First bleed the sick person, then let him or her drink plentifully of the following decoction. Take pearl barley, raisins, and figs, of each two ounces, stick liquorice bruised, half an ounce; boil them in four quarts of water, till it comes to two quarts; strain it for use, and add a quarter of an ounce of salt prunella. You must purge often after this disorder, and the diet must be light.

CURE FOR THE WHITE SWELLING, OR ANY ULCER.

Take two hatsful of the bark of mountain birch, one large burdock root, or two if small; bruise the roots and bark, and put the same in a large iron pot that will hold seven or eight gallons filled with water, which boil until reduced to three; then take out the roots and bark, and put the decoction in a jug, and take a pint every morning fasting, and half a pint two or three times besides, every day.

N.B.—The person is to eat no sauce meat, nor any thing salt; if milk, it must be old and half water, and his constant drink sassafras tea.

A PREPARATION TO WASH THE SORE.

Take two handsful of ivy leaves boiled in three quarts of water till reduced to two, then take out the leaves and put in one quart of water more, and take the inside bark of ash burnt to ashes, put in four spoonsful of the ashes, which boil again; then let it settle, and pour off the liquid, which bottle up for use, and wash the sore twice a day.

WHITE SWELLING.

ANOTHER.—Take a quantity of the blacker kind of shoemake root, scrape off the outside black, then peel off the inner bark, and boil in milk until the root is soft; mash it up, and thicken it with rye meal to the consistence of a poultice, and apply.

CURE FOR A CANCER.
From a Philadelphia Paper.

Take the narrow-leafed dock-root, and boil it in water till it be quite soft; then bathe the part affected in the decoction as hot as can be borne, three or four times a day; the root must then be mashed and applied as a poultice.

This root has proved an effectual cure in many instances. It was first introduced by an Indian woman, who came to the house of a person in the country, who was much afflicted with a cancer in her mouth; the Indian, perceiving something was the matter, inquired what it was, and, on being informed, said she could cure her. The woman consented to a trial, though with little hope of success, having previously used many things without receiving any benefit. The Indian went out, and soon returned with a root, which she boiled and applied as above, and in a short time a cure was effected. The Indian was very careful to conceal what these roots were, and refused giving any information respecting them: but happening one day to lay some of them down, and step out, the woman concealed one of the roots, which she planted, and soon discovered what it was. Not long after, a person in that neighbourhood being afflicted with the same complaint in her face, she informed her of this remedy, and in two weeks she was perfectly cured. Some time ago a man was cured of a confirmed cancer in the back of his hand: after suffering much, and unable to get any rest, being told of this root, it was procured and prepared for him; he kept his hand in the water as hot as he could bear it, for some time; the root was then applied as a poultice, and that night he slept comfortably, and in two weeks his hand was entirely cured.

CURE FOR THE FEVER AND AGUE.

The following simple receipt has never been known to fail, and is now published for the benefit of such as may be suffering under this disagreeable complaint: One ounce yellow Peruvian bark, quarter of an ounce cream of tartar, one tablespoonful pulverized cloves, and one pint Teneriffe wine. Mix them all together; shake it well, and take a wine-glassful every two hours after the fever is off.

N. B.—Before taking the above, a dose of Epsom salts, or other medicine, should be administered to cleanse the stomach, and render the cure more speedy and certain.

ANOTHER.—Just before going to bed, let the patient take off his clothes, and stand under a sieve suspended by a line; let a person pour into the sieve a pail of water fresh from the spring, the shock will be considerable; but let the person wipe dry and go into bed. The effect will be pleasing. It seldom fails curing at three times bathing; often with one.

CURE FOR POISON, BY NEGRO CESAR,

For the discovery of which, the Assembly of South Carolina purchased his freedom, and gave him an annuity of one hundred pounds.

Take roots of plantain and wild hoarhound, fresh or dried, three ounces each; boil them together in two quarts of water, down to one quart, and strain it. Of this decoction let the patient take one-third part three mornings successively, on a fasting stomach, from which, if he finds any relief, it must be continued until he is perfectly recovered. On the contrary, if he finds no alteration after the third dose, it is a sign that the patient has not been poisoned at all, or that it has been with such poison as Cesar's antidote will not remedy—so he may leave off the decoction.

During the cure the patient must live on spare diet, and abstain from eating mutton, pork, butter, or any other fat or oily food.

N. B.—The plantain or hoarhound will either of them cure alone, but they are more efficacious together.

In summer, you may take one handful of the roots

and branches of each, in place of three ounces of the roots of each.

For Drink during the Cure.

Take of the roots of golden rod, six ounces, or in summer, two large handsful of the roots and branches together, and boil them in two quarts of water, down to one quart, to which also may be added a little hoarhound and sassafras; to this decoction, after it is strained, add a glass of rum or brandy, and sweeten it with sugar for ordinary drink. Sometimes an inward fever attends such as are poisoned, for which he orders the following:—

Take one pint of wood-ashes, and three pints of water, stir and mix them well together; let them stand all night, and strain off the ley in the morning, of which ten ounces may be taken, six mornings running, warmed or cold, according to the weather.

These medicines have no sensible operation, though sometimes they work in the bowels, and give a gentle stool.

Symptoms attending such as are Poisoned.

A pain in the breast, difficulty of breathing, a load at the pit of the stomach, an irregular pulse, burning and violent pains of the viscera above and below the navel, very restless at night, sometimes wandering pains over the whole body, a retching inclination to vomit, profuse sweats (which prove always serviceable), slimy stools, both when costive and loose, the face of a pale yellow colour, sometimes a pain and inflammation of the throat; the appetite is generally weak, and some cannot eat any; those who have been long poisoned, are generally very feeble and weak in their limbs; sometimes spit a great deal; the whole skin peels, and likewise the hair falls off.

CURE FOR THE SCARLET FEVER.

We find in the Northampton Courier, a communication from an old physician, in which he gives what he believes to be a sure remedy for this malignant disease. He says a solution of tartar emetic, five grains to a pint of hot water, should be given to the patient, in quantities just sufficient to nauseate, when the febrile symptoms run high. When thirsty, he may drink pretty freely of saffron, or imperial tea. In the use of cathartics, great care should be taken to administer mild medicines, and by all means to avoid the use of calomel. When the patient is troubled with spasmodic affections, opiates should be administered, elixirs to children, and to adults generally, laudanum, to prevent the virus (produced by the exhalations from the body) from being re-absorbed, and thus finding its way back to the lungs, and *vice versa*. I have found the following mode of treatment very beneficial, viz: to wash the patient with milk and water once in five or six hours, and cover with a coat of Indian meal. The writer says, when he was in practice fifty years ago, if he lost one patient in twenty he attributed it to bad management on the part of the nurse, and for thirty years he was uniformly successful whenever he prevailed. We hope this remedy will be found as successful now as it was fifty years ago; but it is possible the disorder has changed in some of its features within half a century. It is now a dreadful scourge to the young, and if a remedy can be found for it, the discoverer will be entitled to the gratitude of the world.

PREVENTIVE FOR SCARLET FEVER.
From the Baltimore American.

As this intractable disease, in its most malignant form, has extensively prevailed during the past winter, and still continues its progress in our city, causing many tears to flow from agonized parents, who have had their darling little ones suddenly snatched from them by its ruthless grasp, I would call the attention of those, whose homes have not yet been made desolate by its inroads, to the following prophylactic or preventive measure, which, among practitioners of medicine in Germany, has been used with such eminent success, but which in this country, I believe, is scarcely known out of the profession.

Dissolve three grains of the extract of Belladonna in one ounce of cinnamon water (triturated together in a mortar), and of this solution give three drops in a little sugar and water, to a child one year old, once a day, increasing the dose one drop for every additional year in the age of the patient. In this minute dose it can do no possible injury; whilst the mass of evidence in favor of its complete prophylactic power, is conclusive.

Impelled by a desire to stay the further progress of this fatal epidemic, it would afford me much satisfaction to have the above information disseminated, and it would be subserving the cause of humanity, to allow it a corner in the columns of your valuable sheet.

MEDICUS.

BALTIMORE, *March* 23, 1844.

CURE FOR CONSUMPTION.

I will not positively say the following remedy is capable of completely eradicating this disorder, but I will venture to affirm, that by a temperate mode of living (avoiding spirituous liquors wholly), wearing flannel next to the skin, and taking every morning half a pint of new milk, mixed with the expressed juice of green hoarhound, the complaint will not only be relieved, but the individual shall procure to himself a length of days beyond what the mildest fever could give room to hope for.

I am myself a living witness of the beneficial effects of this agreeable, and, though innocent, yet powerful application. Four weeks' use of the hoarhound and milk relieved the pains of my breast; enabled me to breathe deep, long, and free; strengthened and harmonized my voice; and restored me to a better state of health than I had enjoyed for many years.

ANOTHER.—Take three quarts of good spring water, a quart of wheat bran, and half a pint of honey; simmer them gently for two or three hours in a stone pot over a slow fire. Let the compound cool sufficiently to admit yeast through it; then put in half a pint of good yeast, and let it stand thirty-six hours. Take half a wine-glass three times a day, a few minutes before eating. If this appears too much, take a less quantity. To the use of this, the subscriber confidently ascribes his rescue from an early grave, to which he was evidently fast hastening, by a consumption brought on by the measles.

R. GILBERT.

A VALUABLE

COLLECTION OF RECEIPTS

FOR THE

CURE OF DISEASES AND COMMON DISTEMPERS,

INCIDENT TO

HORSES, CATTLE, CALVES, SWINE, SHEEP, ETC.

COLLECTED FROM SOME OF THE BEST LATE AUTHORS. ALSO,
CLOSING WITH A FEW BRIEF HINTS FOR THE WINTER.

WITH AN INDEX.

RECEIPTS

FOR

THE CURE OF DISEASES IN BEASTS.

HOW TO FORM A JUDGMENT OF THE AGE OF A HORSE BY HIS TEETH.

At two years old the horse sheds the two middle teeth of the under jaw. At three years old he sheds two other teeth, one on each side of those he shed the year before. At four years old he sheds the two remaining, or corner teeth. At five years old the two middle teeth are full, no longer hollow as all the others are, and the teeth have penetrated the gums. At six years old the four middle teeth are full, the corner teeth only remaining hollow; the tusks are sharp, with the sides fluted. At seven years old the corner teeth are full, the tusks longer and thicker, and the horse is said to be aged.

Note.—It is not meant that exactly at the period above mentioned these changes take place in the horse: much depends upon his constitution, whether he be a late or early foal: also upon the manner in which he has been reared, as to food and shelter, &c. The corner tooth, too, might remain a little hollow after the age of seven, but the appearance is still very unlike the mere shells which they are at the age of six.

AGE OF SHEEP

May be known by examining the front teeth. They are eight in number, and appear during the first year of a small size. In the second year the two middle ones fall out, and their place is supplied by two new teeth, which are easily distinguished by their being of a larger size. In the third year, the two other small teeth, one from each side, drop out, and are replaced by two larger ones; so that there are four large teeth in the middle, and two pointed ones on each side. In the fourth year, the large teeth are six in number, and only two small ones remain, one at each end of the range. In the fifth year, the remaining small teeth are lost, and the whole front teeth are larger. In the sixth year, the whole begin to be worn; and in the seventh, sometimes sooner, some fall out or are broken.

TO PREVENT HORSES BEING TEASED BY FLIES.

Take two or three small handsful of walnut leaves, upon which pour two or three quarts of cold water; let it infuse one night, and pour the whole next morning into a kettle, and let it boil for a quarter of an hour. When cold it will be fit for use. No more is required than to moisten a sponge, and before the horse goes out of the stable, let those parts which are most irritable be smeared over with the liquor, viz: between and upon the ears, the neck and flank, &c. Not only the lady or gentleman who rides out for pleasure will derive benefit from the walnut leaves thus prepared, but the coachman, the wagoner, and all who use horses during the hot months.

SORE TONGUE IN HORSES—A PRETTY CERTAIN CURE.

Dissolve two ounces of copperas, and two of alum,

in a pint of strong vinegar; swab the mouth and tongue with the solution until the disease is removed: then dissolve honey and alum in vinegar, and use it in the same way to heal the tongue.

ANOTHER.—Make a strong decoction of red oak bark, and dissolve a small quantity of alum and copperas, when cold; and then wash the tongue or pour the liquid in the mouth with a bottle, holding it a while, and let the horse throw it out.

LINIMENT FOR THE GALLED BACKS OF HORSES.

KEATING, in his expedition to the source of St. Peter's River, says:—For the information of other travellers, we may mention, that, after having tried many applications to the backs of horses, when galled, we have found none that succeeded so well as white lead moistened with milk. When milk was not to be procured, oil was substituted. Whenever the application was made in the early stage of the wound, we have found it to be very effectual, and it is likewise a convenient one, as two ounces of white lead sufficed for the whole of our party for more than a month.

SADDLE GALLS.

Saddle galls are generally occasioned by an unequal pressure of the saddle, or by a saddle being badly fitted to a horse's back, and if neglected they grow into very ugly and troublesome sores. When these inflamed tumors are first discovered, cold water alone is frequently sufficient to disperse and drive them away, if applied as soon as the saddle is pulled off; but when that will not have the desired effect, the back may be washed twice a day in a mixture of sharp vinegar, one gill; spirits of any kind, one gill;

sweet oil or fresh butter, one tablespoonful; to be well mixed before used.

SWELLINGS ON HORSES OR CATTLE.

To scatter swellings on horses or cattle, take two quarts of proof whiskey, or other proof spirits; warm it over coals, but not to blaze; dissolve in it a pint of soft soap; when cool put it in a bottle, and add one ounce of camphor. When dissolved it will form the liquid opodeldoc, and is then ready for application, forming a cheap and useful remedy. When the swelling is on the leg, or any part that will receive a bandage, such bandage should be applied, and wet with the opodeldoc.

KING'S OIL FOR CURING WOUNDS ON HORSES AND CATTLE.

One ounce of green copperas, two ounces of white vitriol, two ounces of common salt, two ounces of linseed oil, and eight ounces of molasses; pulverize the copperas, and boil all over a slow fire fifteen minutes in a pint of wine; when almost cold add one ounce oil of vitriol, and four ounces spirit of turpentine. Apply to the wound, with a quill or feather, which will immediately set the wound to running, and perform a certain cure.

Mr. Tucker,—As there are many useful receipts hidden from the public, for the sake of speculation in a small way, by many who would be thought something of in the world, I am induced to lay before the public the above receipt for making king's oil, so called, which perhaps excels any other for the cure of wounds on horses or cattle, and which has long been known only by a few persons. Feeling a desire to contribute to the good of the public, but more especially to the farmers of Genesee, I send you the above valuable receipt for publication.

STEPHEN PALMER.

Middlebury, Dec. 10, 1834.

CRACKS IN THE HEELS, OR WOUNDS IN HORSES.

Sugar of lead two drachms; white vitriol, one drachm; a strong infusion of red oak bark, or elm, all well mixed together. Wash or bathe the parts affected with the above preparation.

LOST APPETITE IN A HORSE.

Horses lose their appetites from various causes, viz. :—excessive fatigue, want of a change in food, dirty fodder, mouldy corn, or a dirty manger, &c., but most frequently by the approach of some disease. So soon as you discover a horse has lost his appetite, observe the following treatment, viz. :—take from the neck vein half a gallon of blood; take of asafœtida, a quarter of an ounce; salt, one tablespoonful; sassafras tea, one quart; mix and give them a drench. On the second day, take of glauber salts, one pound; warm water one quart; after dissolving the salts give it as a drench, and in two or three days the appetite will be restored, unless the animal is labouring under some disease, which may be ascertained by the symptoms.

ANOTHER.—Take half a pound of saltpetre, half a pound of alum, and half a pound alum salt; pulverize and mix them well together, and every eight or ten days give the horse a tablespoonful in his food; his coat, flesh, and spirits will soon reward his master for his care.

MASH FOR HORSES.

A mash is generally given to a horse for the purpose of cooling the system, opening the bowels, and for disguising different kinds of medicine, which may be necessary to be administered, which, if given in any other way, would be attended with difficulty, and would be unproductive of effects so salutary.

Mash No 1. Take of bran, one gallon; sassafras tea (scalding hot), one quart; powdered brimstone, one tablespoonful; saltpetre, one teaspoonful.

No. 2. Take oats, one gallon; flour of sulphur, one tablespoonful; saltpetre, one teaspoonful; boiling water, one quart.

No. 3. Take of bran, one gallon; glauber salts, four ounces; sulphur, one tablespoonful; sassafras tea (scalding hot), one quart. Let them be well mixed, and given milk-warm, not permitting the horse to drink cold water for six hours afterward.

CURIOUS CASE OF FARRIER.

Some time ago a very valuable mare, belonging to Mr. C. Limy, of Boylin, was gored by a bull, and the entrails protruded through the wound.

As there appeared no possible remedy, the animal was left in the field to die, when a neighbouring man, named Moran, undertook to cure her. After returning the entrails and sewing up the wound, he procured a large piece of sheet lead, placed it over the spot, and afterward drew the skin across it, and sewed it up. After an interval of some days, he again opened the skin, and removed the lead, when the wound appeared completely healed. The skin was a second time sewed up; and in less than a month after, the animal was able to plough as well as ever.

BLISTERS.

Previous to the application of a blister to any part

of a horse, the hair should either be shaved or cut off as close as possible; the blistering ointment should be regularly spread with a warm knife on a stout piece of osnaburg; and during the operation of the blister, the horse should be tied short to prevent his biting the part, or doing other injury.

Blister No. 1. Take of Spanish flies, half an ounce; oil of turpentine, one ounce; hog's lard, four ounces; mix them well, and the blister is ready for use.

No. 2. Take of tar, four ounces; vitriolic acid, two drachms; oil of origanum, half an ounce; hog's lard, two ounces; Spanish flies, two ounces. This blister is excellent for the spavin.

CLYSTER, OR GLYSTER.

As clysters very often are the means of saving horses' lives, I shall here recommend the best and simplest method of administering them. Take a large bladder, cut off the neck, and soften it in warm water. Take a pewter pipe, common reed, or any other smooth tube, nine or ten inches long, and not more than an inch in diameter; the clyster must then be poured through a funnel into the bag, and securely tied around one end of the tube; the other must be made perfectly smooth and rounded, well oiled, and introduced into the anus several inches; the liquor in the bladder must be forced through the tube by pressure with the hand. When a clyster is given, a horse should be placed with his head down hill, and if he refuses to stand, a twitch should be put upon his nose.

Clysters are of three kinds—opening, anodyne, and nourishing. For the first purpose take a gallon of warm water, with from half a pound to a pound of common salt dissolved in it; to which add four or five ounces of linseed oil. For the second take two drachms of solid opium, dissolve them, or rather mix them well with about half a pint of warm water, and add from a quart to three pints of Indian meal, or wheat flour gruel. For the third purpose, rich broths, wheat flour gruel, and other nourishing fluids, are recommended.

With respect to the first kind of clysters, it may be observed that gruel is commonly preferred to warm water; but, according to my experience, the latter does just as well as the former. As to the second, tincture of opium may be substituted for solid opium, and is by some preferred to it; but the quantity should not exceed two ounces, on account of the spirit in which this opium is dissolved. The third kind of clyster is required only in lock-jaw, or in diseases of the throat which prevent swallowing, and in these its utility seems to be very questionable.

As soon as the clyster has been injected, the tail should be kept close to the fundament for a few minutes, to prevent its being too hastily returned. This is particularly necessary when the anodyne clyster has been employed. The pipe must be oiled, or greased before it is introduced, and if its passage be obstructed by hard dung lodged in the gut, the hand should be gradually introduced in order to remove it.

CURE FOR THE SCOURS IN HORSES.

Put into a junk bottle one pint of good gin, and one ounce of indigo; shake well together, and pour it down him.—I have known it from personal observation to have the desired effect, and complete a cure in a short time.—*Yankee Farmer.*

COLIC IN HORSES.

Jamestown seed, from 4 to 10 tablespoonsful, boiled, and poured off, given to a horse, will effect a cure in 10 or 15 minutes. Bleed the horse in the mouth.

ANOTHER.—Make and give him a drench composed of a tablespoonful of strong mustard dissolved in a pint of water; which may be administered in a black junk bottle, by raising the horse's head a sufficient height. If it be uncertain when the horse was taken, as in that case there will be danger of inflammation, on discovery of the disorder, bleed a vein immediately. The remedy here described, is said to be immediate and infallible.

ANOTHER.—I was lately told by a gentleman of Prince George county, that a teacupful of spirits of turpentine would give instant relief to horses laboring under this disorder. He added that, on one occasion, all the oxen of two of his carts were hoven—that is, as you know, suddenly swollen by the generation of gas in the stomach, from eating green food. The overseer expected all would die, when our informant ordered a teacupful of spirits of turpentine, diffused in oil, to be given to each. The relief was in every case instantaneous and effectual, almost before he could have thought there was time to swallow. Such facts should always be communicated for wide diffusion and preservation.—*American Farmer.*

COLIC, OR GRIPES.

Symptoms.—The symptoms of the colic commence with great restlessness and uneasiness in the horse's manner of standing; frequently he paws, voids small quantities of excrement, and makes many fruitless attempts to stale; kicks his belly with his hind legs;

often looks round to his flanks, groaning, expressive of the pain he feels; lies down, rolls, gets up again and sometimes for a moment appears to find relief. But the pain soon returns with double violence; his ears are generally cold, and he often sweats about the flank and shoulders; his body swells, and he frequently shows a disposition to lie down in great haste.

A TABLE FOR DISTINGUISHING

Between the Colic, or Gripes, and Inflammation of the bowels of horses, by the symptoms that mark the character of each.

SPASMODIC OR FLATULENT COLIC.	INFLAMMATION OF THE BOWELS.
1. Pulse natural, though sometimes a little lower. (1.)	1. Pulse very quick and small. (2.)
2. The horse lies down and rolls upon his back.	2. He lies down and suddenly rises up again, seldom rolling upon his back.
3. The legs and ears are generally warm.	3. Legs and ears generally cold.
4. Attacks suddenly, is never preceded, and seldom accompanied, by any symptoms of fever.	4. In general attacks gradually, is commonly preceded, and always accompanied by symptoms of fever.
5. There are frequently short intermissions.	5. No intermissions can be observed.

(1.) Pulse natural.—When in health, the pulsations or strokes are from thirty-six to forty in a minute; those of large heavy horses being slower than those of smaller; and those of old ones slower than those of young animals. When either are just off a quick pace, the strokes increase in number; as they do if he be alarmed or animated by the familiar cry of the hounds.

(2.) Pulse very quick and small.—Fever of the simple or common kind usually increases the pulsations to double the healthy number, as the fever increases in violence, and particularly in cases of inflammation of the bowels, the pulse beats still higher, and reaches to a hundred in a minute or more. To ascertain either state, the attendant should apply the points of his fingers gently to the artery which lies nearest the surface. Some prefer consulting the temporal artery, which is situated about an inch and a half backward from the corner of the eye. Others again, and they are the greatest number, think it best to feel it underneath the edge of the jaw-bone, where the facial artery passes on under the skin only to the side of the face. In either case, too great pressure would stop the pulsation altogether; though by so trying the artery against the jaw-bone, will prove whether it be in such a rigid state of excitement as attends high fever; or elastic and springy, slipping readily from under the finger, as it does when health prevails, and the strokes follow each other regularly. The presence of high fever is farther indicated by a kind of twang, or vibration, given by the pulse against the finger points, resembling such as would be felt were we to take hold of a distended whip cord or wire between the fingers and cause it to vibrate like a fiddle string, sharply; whereas, in health, a swell is felt in the vibration as if the string were made of soft materials, and less straightened. Languid or slow pulse, and scarcely perceptible in some of the beats or strokes, indicates lowness of spirits, debility, or being used up : if languor be felt at intervals only, a few strokes being very quick, and then again a few very slow, this indicates low fever, in which bleeding would do no harm, &c.—*A. Turf. R. & S. Mag.*

Remedies.—No. 1. Take from the neck vein half a gallon of blood; take of laudanum one ounce, or mint tea one quart, milk warm; mix them well in a bottle, and give the contents as a drench; let the horse be well rubbed under the belly, and prepare and give an injection of meal, water, molasses, salt, and hog's lard, milk warm.

No. 2. Take of mint tea one and a half pints; gin, or any spirituous liquor, half a pint; mix them well in a bottle, and give them as a drench, taking care to rub the horse well. Should it not have the desired effect in fifteen minutes, repeat the dose.

No. 3. Take of camphor a quarter of an ounce, oil of turpentine half an ounce, mint tea one pint; mix them in a bottle and give them as a drench; confine the horse in a close stable, cover him with three or four blankets, and under his belly place a large tub of boiling water, which will readily throw him into a profuse sweat, and relieve him from pain.

No. 4. In addition to the above, clysters ought to be administered by injecting the following ingredients, viz. : water, half a gallon; salt, one handful; oil of any kind, one pint; molasses, one pint; mix the whole and inject it; and repeat it every half hour, until the bowels are well opened.

FOUNDER IN HORSES.

A founder evidently proceeds from surfeit; a horse ridden until heated and fatigued, and fed too plentifully while warm and hungry, and swallowing his food too greedily that he may lie down and rest his wearied limbs while the stable is wet or damp, and the horse in a copious sweat, are the best reasons that can be given for the formation of the disease. Instead of rising up refreshed, the poor animal is stiff and useless. If he had got leave to cool perfectly, and been fed sparingly, he would have escaped this sore complaint.

The cure is a lump of alum, the size of a walnut, reduced to powder and dissolved in warm water; the horse must be drenched with this liquid, which in a short time will throw him into a profuse perspiration, and he will be able to pursue his journey the next day, and if not badly foundered, in a few hours.

ANOTHER.—So soon as you are convinced that your horse is foundered, take from his neck vein at least one gallon of blood; give a drench of one quart of strong sassafras tea, one teaspoonful of saltpetre, and a quarter of an ounce of asafœtida, and do not permit him to eat or drink for five or six hours; at the expiration of which time, should he not be evidently better, repeat the bleeding, taking half a gallon of blood, and give another drench: at night, offer him some bran or oats, scalded with sassafras tea, and if it can be procured, let him have green food fresh from the field, for it has the happy effect of opening the bowels, and cooling the system. His feet should be nicely cleansed out, and stuffed with fresh cow manure; his drink should be at least one half sassafras tea, with a small handful of salt thrown in. By the morning, should the horse be better, nothing farther is necessary, only being careful not to overfeed him. But should there be no change for the better, tie a small cord just above his knees, and with a lancet or fleam bleed him in a vein that runs around the coronet just above the hoof. Take from each leg a pint of blood; give a pound of salts dissolved in three half pints of water, in form of a drench; keep his feet stuffed with fresh cow manure, and bathe his legs with equal parts of sharp vinegar, spirits, and sweet oil or lard. By attention to these directions, in two or three days the horse will again be fit for use.

ANOTHER.—When a horse is slightly foundered, take a gill of spirits of turpentine, and one pint of whiskey, and drench him with it: when he sweats, rub him down well, and nothing more need be required. For a severe founder, drench him with a quart of melted lard, which is said to be an effectual cure.

ANOTHER.—I send you the following prescription, which you may give a place in your useful paper, if you think it will be any advantage to planters and travellers.

As soon as you find your horse is foundered, bleed him in the neck, in proportion to the greatness of the founder. In extreme cases you may bleed him as long as he can stand up. Then give him a strong drench of salt and water. Be careful not to let him drink too much water afterwards. Then anoint around the edges of his hoofs with spirits of turpentine, and your horse will be well in one hour.

A founder pervades every part of the system of a horse. The phlegms arrest it from the blood; the salt and water arrest it from the stomach and bowels; and the spirits of turpentine arrest it from the feet and limbs.

I once rode a hired horse ninety miles in two days, returning him at night the second day; and his owner would not have known that he had been foundered if I had not told him, and his founder was one of the deepest kind.

I once, in a travel of seven hundred miles, foundered my horse three times, and I do not think that my journey was retarded more than one day by the misfortune, having in all the cases practised in the above prescription. I have known a foundered horse turned in at night on green food; in the morning he would be well, having been purged by the green food. All founders must be attended to immediately.

South Western Farmer.

ANOTHER.—If your horse founders over night, in the morning take a pint of hog's lard, put it in a vessel, and make it boiling hot; clean his hoofs well, and set his foot in the lard. Heat it for each foot boiling hot; take a spoon and put the fat over the hoof, as near the hair as possible, and if this be done early in the morning he will be fit for use in three hours after. It is better to remove the horse's shoes.

MALANDERS ON HORSES.

It consists of chops, or cracks on the inside of the fore leg, against the knee, discharging a red, sharp humour. To cure this disease, wash the cracks with warm soap suds, or old wine; then rub them twice a day with an ointment of hog's lard, mixed with two drachms sublimate of mercury; or apply a poultice of the roots of marsh mallows, flax-seed, softened with linseed oil, tying it on with a roller. Continue that till the seeds fall off, and the sores become clean; afterwards a mixture of turpentine and quicksilver will be a proper application.

REMEDY FOR THE HEAVES IN HORSES.

Take half a pound of good ginger for a horse; give two tablespoonsful a day; one in the morning and the other in the evening; mix with wheat bran. This receipt has been selling for five hundred dollars at the Eastward, where the efficacy of the above medicine has been proved.

CURE FOR COUGH IN HORSES.

Half a pound of nitre, a quarter of a pound of black

regulus of antimony, two ounces of antimony; mix well in a mortar, and make it up into doses of one ounce each; give the horse one dose in a cold mash, mixed every night in mild weather for three nights. Then omit it for a week. If he does not get better of his cough, repeat it. Care is necessary that the animal should not be exposed while warm to stand in a cold wind; otherwise exercise him gently, and treat him as usual.

A BROKEN-WINDED HORSE.

It is easy to discover a broken-winded horse. By giving him a little brisk exercise he will draw up his flanks, and drop them suddenly, breathe with great difficulty, and make a disagreeable wheezing noise. The seat of the disease appears, from dissection, to be in the lungs; the heart and lungs being found of twice their natural size, which prevents their performing their office with ease, in the action of respiration. Broken wind is sometimes produced in a horse by excessive fatigue, heavy draughts, sudden changes from heat to cold, and other cruel treatment. It would be advisable to dispose of such horses at any price, as they are not worth their feeding. This complaint, I believe, does not admit of a perfect cure: but by much care they may be greatly relieved. The food should be compact and nutritious, such as corn and old hay. Carrots are excellent in this case, also parsnips and beets, probably on account of the saccharine matter they contain. I have heard that molasses has been given in the water (which should be in very small quantities), with very great success. Some have used tar water, others praise the effects of lime-water; but the greatest dependence should be in very sparing supplies of substantial food. The exercise should be regular, but never beyond a walking pace. If the symptomatic cough be troublesome, take away about three quarts of blood every other day.

ANOTHER.—This disorder is caused by overfeeding, by violent exercise when the horse is too full, or by letting a horse go into water when he is too hot and sweaty; or, it frequently originates from an obstinate cold, not well cured. The only remedy we have known to prove efficient, is to feed a horse on good, healthy food—corn, and not much hay, or feed him upon potatoes, and whenever water is given him it should be impregnated with saltpetre and sal ammoniac. Lime water, freely given, has in many instances cured this complaint.

THUMPS IN HORSES.

Thumps are caused by overheating and fast riding or driving. Take one pint of brandy or good whiskey, beat up a quarter of a pound of black pepper, mix it and drench him. Or take a dozen eggs, hold up his head and break them and put them down his throat shell and all, and he will recover immediately.

WIND GALLS.

Wind galls are spongy and flatulent humours that make their appearance on both sides of the legs, just above the pastern joint or fetlock. It is seldom that a horse is found entirely clear of them; particularly about the hind legs, if he be much used.

They are produced by hard usage, strains, bruies, &c., of the back, sinews, or the sheath that covers them, which, by being overstretched, have some of their fibres ruptured: whence may ooze out the fluid which is commonly found with the included air.

When wind galls make their first appearance, they are easily cured by a bath and bandage. Boil red oak bark to a strong decoction, add some sharp vinegar and a little alum, let the parts be fomented twice a day, warm as the hand can be held in it; then take a woollen cloth, dip it in the bath, and bind the ankle up as tight as possible, without giving pain to the horse.

Should this method not succeed after a thorough trial, the swelled or puffed parts may be opened with a sharp knife, but blistering with flies is less dangerous, and generally attended with equal success.

Wind galls give to a horse a gouty and clumsy appearance; but I have never known lameness produced by them, or any other injury, except that of stiffening his legs as he advances in years. They furnish strong proof that the animal has rendered much service.

SITFAST ON HORSES.

Sitfast proceeds from the part being frequently bruised with a saddle until it becomes extremely hard, and after remaining some length of time is not unlike a horny substance. A cure cannot be performed unless the knife is used for the purpose of cutting it entirely out, after which the fresh wound can be healed with the greatest ease in a very short time, by using either of the following mixtures:—

No. 1. Take of brandy half a pint, honey half a pint, alum two ounces.

No. 2. Take of blue stone a quarter of an ounce; spirits of turpentine two tablespoonsful; spring water one pint.

No. 3. Take of sugar of lead, half an ounce; alum, one ounce; copperas, half an ounce. Let the ingredients be well mixed, and the sitfast washed twice a day. After the wound is washed, clean with soap and water.

SCRATCHES.

The scratches is a disease which soon places a horse in such a situation as to render him unfit for any kind of service. When it is permitted to run upon a horse for a length of time without any remedy being applied, the ankles and legs swell very much, and lameness is produced in so great a degree that he is scarcely able to move.

The scratches are produced from many different causes, as hard riding, dirty stables, legs left wet at night without being rubbed, standing on his own manure or mud in the stall where he is confined, &c. Although much inflammation may appear, and the disease discover much inveteracy, the cure is not difficult.

Remedies.—No. 1. Remove the horse to a clean stall ; with strong soap suds wash his legs and ankles nicely ; clean out his feet ; then wash every inflamed part or sore in strong copperas water twice a day until the cure is performed. Take half a gallon of blood from the neck vein, and give a mash twice a week, of one gallon of bran, one teaspoonful of saltpetre, and one tablespoonful of powdered brimstone. Great attention should be paid to the cleanliness of the stable.

No. 2. After the horse is placed in a clean stall, and his legs and ankles nicely washed with warm soap suds, take of blue stone, one ounce ; of alum, four ounces ; to which add half a gallon of strong decoction of red oak bark ; stir them together, until the alum and blue stone are dissolved ; then wash the cracks, sores, or inflamed parts twice a day, and the cure will be effected in a very short time. Light or green food would be preferable to any other for a horse thus diseased, until the cure is performed.

No. 3. After washing the legs and ankles clean with soap suds, take flour of sulphur or powdered brimstone, one tablespoonful; mix them well together, and anoint the sores and parts inflamed twice a day. A horse will get well much sooner when confined in a clean stall than by running at large.

No. 4. Boil poke root to a strong decoction, and bathe the ankles twice a day. In all cases a clean stable will aid you much in making a quick cure of the scratches.

ANOTHER.—This disorder or difficulty is too well known to all that own these noble animals, or deal in them, to need a particular description of mine. The remedy is simple, safe, and certain in all cases which have come to my knowledge, however inveterate. It is only to mix white lead and linseed oil, in such proportions as will render the application convenient; and I have never known more than two or three applications necessary completely to effect a cure.

ANOTHER.

To the Editor of the American Farmer.

For each dose, take a handful of the roots of dwarf ash, known in some places by the name of "old man's beard," the Germans call it "noodle tree," from the circumstance of its having a beautiful white bloom covering the whole top, and hanging in the form of tassels; in the spring it resembles the common ash, but in this country it is a dwarf. I never saw it more than six or eight feet high. Chop the roots small, put in two quarts of water, and boil down to about half its quantity. Give this dose every other day until you have given three, then bleed freely in the neck—a small quantity of lard or neat's foot oil may be applied externally to soften the sore. For a desperate case, the operation should be repeated. I never saw but one case in which it was necessary to give the second operation. It is best to bleed copiously.

JONATHAN BEARD.
Midway, N. C,. 1843.

REMEDY FOR THE POLL EVIL, OR FISTULA IN HORSES.

When the swelling breaks, or if it has been some time a running sore, it will have a pipe or tube, from which the matter discharges; into this crowd a lump of pearlash, or potash, as large as you can, with your finger. Three such applications will cure the worst case.

ANOTHER.—From a horse's rubbing and sometimes striking his poll against the lower edge of the manger, or hanging back in the stall, and bruising the part with the halter, or from the frequent and painful stretchings of the ligaments and muscles by unnecessary tight reigning, and occasionally, we fear, from a violent blow on the poll, carelessly or wantonly inflicted, inflammation comes on, and a swelling appears, hot, tender, and painful. We have just stated, that the ligament of the neck passes over the atlas, or first bone, without being attached to it; and the seat of inflammation is between the ligament and the bone beneath; and being thus situated, it is serious in its nature, and difficult of treatment. The first thing to be attempted, is to abate the inflammation by bleeding, physic, and the application of cold lotions to the part; by these means the tumor will sometimes be dispersed. This system, however, must not be pursued too far. If the swelling increases, and the heat and tenderness likewise increase, matter will form in the tumor; and then our object will be to hasten its formation by warm fomentations, poultices or stimulating embrocations. As soon as matter is formed, which may be known by the softness of the tumor, and before it has time to spread around and eat into the neighbouring parts, it should be evacuated. And now comes the art of poll evil : the openings into the tumor must be so contrived that all the matter shall run out, and continue to run out as it is formed, and not collect at the bottom of the ulcer, irritating and corroding it. This can be effected by a seton alone. The needle should enter at the top of the tumor, penetrate through its bottom, and be brought out at the side of the neck, a little below the abscess, without anything more than this, except frequent fomentations with warm water, to keep the part clean, and to obviate inflammation. Poll evil, in its early stage, will frequently be cured. If the ulcer has deepened and spread, and threatens to eat into the ligaments of the joints of the neck, it may be necessary to stimulate its surface, and perhaps painfully so, in order to bring it to a healthy state, and dispose it to fill up; and in extreme cases even the scalding mixture of the farrier may be called into requisition. This, however, will be ineffectual, except the pus or matter is enabled by the use of setons perfectly to run out of the wound : and the application of these setons will require the skill and anatomical knowledge of the veterinary surgeon. In very desperate cases, the wound may not be fairly exposed to the action if our caustic applications, without the division of the ligament of the neck, by which we have described the head as being almost entirely supported. This, however, may be done with perfect safety, for although the ligament is carried on to the occipital bone, and some strength is gained by this prolongation of it, the main strength is on the second bone; and the head will continue to be supported, although the ligament should be divided between the second bone and the head. The divided ligament will soon unite again, and its former usefulness will be restored when the wound is healed.

STAGGERS.

Symptoms.—The symptoms of the staggers are a drowsiness, eyes inflamed, half shut, and full of tears, the appetite bad; the disposition to sleep generally increased, feebleness, a continual hanging of the head, or resting it on the manger; rearing, falling, and being in a state of insensibility; walking a small circle for a considerable length of time; the ears hot, with a burning fever, &c.

REMEDY.—Take from the neck vein half a gallon of blood three times a week; take of sassafras tea three half pints, plantain juice half a pint, asafœtida, half an ounce, saltpetre, one teaspoonful; mix and give them a drink three mornings in a week; give an injection, composed of one pint of meal, two quarts of water, one quart of molasses, and one spoonful of hog's lard; let the horse be moderately exercised, and whenever he is standing he should be well rubbed; give a mash twice a week, composed of one gallon of bran, one tablespoonful of sulphur, one teaspoonful of saltpetre, one quart of boiling sassafras tea, and an eighth of an ounce of asafœtida, not permitting the horse to drink cold water for six hours afterwards. Should he be much mended by this treatment, nothing more will be necessary, except feeding him on bran, or light food of any kind; but should he appear to receive no benefit from these attentions in four or five days, take of calomel twenty-five grains; of opium two drachms; of camphor two drachms; powdered fennel seed, one drachm; of syrup of any kind, a sufficient quantity to make the ingredients into a ball, which may be given every morning for four or five days, by which time the horse will get well, if his disease will admit of cure.

Horses that are confined in a stable never have the staggers; consequently it would be advisable for every person whose situation will admit of it to confine their horses, particularly at night, during the spring and fall months.

BLIND STAGGERS.

This disease appears to be a compression upon the brain, caused by a collection of wind and matter in the forehead. The writer witnessed a cure effected in the following manner :—A hole was bored with a nail gimblet through the skull, on the curl of hair central between the eyes. In various instances he has heard of its being applied with uniform success. This remedy was discovered by an attempt to kill, and thus relieve a horse from the distress of this disease. His skull was fractured by the stroke of an axe. The morning following the horse was found feeding, apparently well. The remedy may be applied by any person, as the horse very soon becomes helpless after the attack, and immediate relief is afforded by letting out the matter, &c.

Those who are too timid to try the above remedy,

may resort to one less severe; and as the writer has understood, from a creditable source, equally successful. Make a vertical incision in the skin between the eyes; separate it from the skull, so as to make a sufficient cavity to contain a gill of salt. A cure very soon will be effected.

FISTULA.

The fistula in the withers generally proceeds from some blow or bruise, and is the most disagreeable disease to which a horse is subject. I would recommend to every person whose situation will admit of the sacrifice to dispose of a horse thus unfortunately affected for whatever sum he would bring, or even give him away, sooner than be at the expense and trouble, and run a risk of performing a cure, which, if completed, would be tedious, and the horse much lessened in value in consequence of being disfigured by the scar which will unavoidably be left. The remedy here recommended is severe, but it will have the desired effect more speedily than any other.

As soon as the fistula assumes a formidable appearance, fomentations of bitter herbs should be employed, such as wormwood, camomile, bay leaves, mullen, life everlasting, &c., boiled in water to a strong decoction, and, after being strained, should be applied hot as the horse can bear it without giving pain, by means of large woollen cloths. This application promotes suppuration; and when matter is formed, let the tumour be opened, so that its contents may be completely evacuated: after which let the sore be nicely washed with strong soap suds, and apply the following ointment once a day:—Take of verdigris half an ounce, oil of turpentine one ounce, copperas half an ounce, ointment of yellow resin four ounces, to be well mixed together. As soon as healthy matter is discharged from the fistula, the ointment may be discontinued, and nothing more will be necessary, except keeping it perfectly clean with soap suds.

When the fistula first makes its appearance, it may be removed or prevented by placing a rowel or seton in each shoulder, just below the swelled or inflamed part, which should be kept running two or three weeks.

FARCY.

To effect a cure in this distressing disease, in its first stage, bleed three times the first week, taking half a gallon of blood at each bleeding; feed principally on bran, oats, or any food easily digested, and the long food green, if to be had; remove all filth from, or about the stable, taking care to keep it neat and clean afterward; give three mashes a week, of bran, scalded with sassafras tea, one tablespoonful of powdered brimstone, and one teaspoonful of saltpetre (not permitting the horse to drink for six hours afterward); take half an ounce of asafœtida, which can be procured in any apothecary's shop, wrap it in a clean linen rag, and nail it in the bottom of the manger in which he is fed: all his drink must be equal quantities of sassafras, boiled in water to a strong decoction, and half an ounce of asafœtida should be placed in his watering bucket, in the same manner as directed for the manger; the buds or ulcers should be washed once a day with blue-stone, or copperas water, and if the knees or ankles are swelled, spread on a piece of buckskin mercurial ointment, and bind them up as tight as possible without giving pain.

The second week bleed twice, taking half a gallon of blood each bleeding, if the horse is in tolerable order; or if poor, only half the quantity: give the same number of mashes as directed for the first week; also the same drink, taking care to renew the asafœtida in the manger and bucket, should it be sufficiently exhausted to require it.

The third week bleed but once, taking one quart of blood: in other respects observe the same treatment as directed for the first and second weeks. The horse should be moderately exercised about a mile twice a day, and occasionally should be offered a little hommony, as change to keep up his appetite. By the time your attentions for the third week expire, if the disease is only local, it will not only be removed, but the plight of the horse will be much improved.

When the farcy begins to make its appearance epidemically, the case is rendered difficult, and will require the aid of more active medicine. Prepare and give to a horse thus diseased a ball every night for a week, composed of twenty-five grains of calomel, a quarter of an ounce of powdered fennel-seed, a small quantity of syrup of any kind, and as much crumb of loaf bread as will make a ball about the size of an English walnut.

All buds or ulcers should be washed clean in bluestone water; after which they should be well rubbed around with mercurial ointment once a day; a narrow pitch plaster should be laid on at the joining of the head and neck, in the direction of the throat-latch, for the purpose of taking off the hair, which will happen in two or three days; after which, a lump of mercurial ointment, about the size of a hickory-nut, must be rubbed on the naked part, among the large glands of the throat, until it is entirely absorbed, every night and morning, until the expiration of the week. Added to which, the treatment generally may be the same as before recommended in the more simple stage of the farcy, with these exceptions: the drink should never be cold, but the air taken off, or milk-warm; the mashes without sulphur counteract the effects of the calomel and ointment: he should not be bled, and great care should be used to prevent his getting wet, and catching cold in any way, while under the course of physic.

At the expiration of the week, stop with the balls and ointment for a week, adding sulphur to the mashes, as directed in the first stage of farcy. At the expiration of the second week, stop with the sulphur, and again commence with the balls and ointment. Go on in this manner, continuing to change the medicine each week, until the cure is performed.

It may sometimes happen that a horse's mouth will become sore before the expiration of a week, when taking the balls and using the ointment. Whenever this is discovered, stop with the balls, and add sulphur to the mashes, which will readily remove the soreness about the mouth.

STRAINS.

Strains, in whatever part of the horse, either produced from running, slips, blows, or hard riding, are the relaxing, overstretching or breaking the muscles or tendinous fibres. A strain, unless uncommonly bad, may be cured in a short time by applying the following remedies:

No. 1. Take of sharp vinegar one pint, spirits of any kind half a pint, camphor one ounce; mix them well together, and bathe the part injured twice a day; a piece of flannel, wet with the mixture, and wrapped around the part, will be very beneficial; take from the neck vein half a gallon of blood.

No. 2. Take of opodeldoc (which can be procured at any apothecary's shop), a piece the size of a marble, and rub it on the strained part with the naked hand twice a day until the hand becomes dry. Should the injured part resist both of these remedies, you may conclude the injury is a very serious one, which nothing but time can relieve, and the horse must be turned out upon grass a sufficient length of time for nature herself to perform the great operation.

RING BONE.

The ring bone partakes of the nature of the spavin, and frequently proceeds from the same cause. It makes its appearance on the lower part of the pastern, and sometimes immediately beyond the coffin joint. It is a hard and bony substance, and generally reaches half round the ankle, which gives to the ankle an unnatural appearance, and causes the horse to go stiff and lame. Its name has proceeded from its resemblance to a ring. It seldom admits of a cure, consequently a horse diseased with it is worth but little. When the ring bone first makes its appearance, blisters of flies have sometimes been employed with success. But after growing to full size, and remaining some length of time, to offer a remedy would be deceitful and inefficient.

REMEDY.—A strong preparation of corrosive sublimate added to Spanish flies and Venice turpentine, and mixed with hog's lard, will often dissolve a ring bone.

SPLINT.

The splint is a hard lump or excrecsence that grows upon the fore legs of a horse, between the fetlock and the knee. It is unpleasant to the eye, but seldom does injury, unless situated on the back of the leg, and immediately under the large tendons, in which case lameness is always produced, and the cure rendered difficult.

When the splint is situated in the usual place, and grows so large as to be unfavorable to beauty, to remove it, bathe the part with hot vinegar twice a day, and have the knot or splint with a smooth round stick, after bathing for ten or fifteen minutes; by the expiration of a week the knot will perceptibly decrease in size, and finally in a short time will disappear but; should such means not have the desired effect, shave off the hair over the lump, and apply a blister of Spanish flies, which in a short time will effectually remove it. The splint, when first making its appearance, will cause a horse to limp a little; and, as he advances in years may stiffen him, and cause him to stumble. But I have never known any serious injury to result from such an excrescence, unless placed beneath the large tendons.

STRING HALT.

The string halt affects horses in their hind legs, and consists in a false action or involuntary use of a muscle which twitches one of the legs almost up to the belly; and sometimes the string halt is produced by a muscle being overstrained, or a violent blow on the hind parts. Good rubbing, and baths of warm vinegar and sweet oil, afford momentary relief, but a permanent cure need not be expected. A horse thus injured is incapable of faithfully performing a journey, although he may be ridden four or five miles without appearing too sick with fatigue. Such a horse is very objectionable, being uneasy to the rider, and must give pain to every person who is in the habit of seeing him ridden.

SPAVIN.

A spavined horse may be considered as one completely ruined; for a permanent cure can rarely be effected, if attempted even on its first appearance.

The spavin is a lump, knot, or swelling, on the inside of the hock, below the joint, that benumbs the limbs, and destroys the free use of the hind legs. It causes a horse to be extremely lame, and to experience, apparently, very excruciating pain.

In the purchase of a horse, great respect should be paid to his bringing up his hind parts well, as a spavined horse never makes a full step with the leg affected; also to the shape of his hocks, in order to discover if there is any knot or unnatural prominence about the joints, which is an evidence of the spavin. When a horse is thus diseased, he is unfit for any kind of service, even the meanest drudgery, being in constant pain, and unable to perform labor. Horses sometimes have the spavin when there is no lump apparent near the joint, the disease being seated in the joint. To detect such spavin, and to prevent a cunning fellow (who may have given the animal rest, blistered and bathed the parts with double distilled spirits, and formed a temporary relief), from imposing on a purchaser, have the horse ridden in three quarters speed, about one mile out and back, occasionally fretting, cracking, and drawing him up suddenly and short; after which, let him be ridden in cold water up to the belly: then place him in a stall, without interruption, for about half an hour, by which time he will be perfectly cool. Then have him led out, and moved gently. If he has received a temporary cure of spavin, he will show lameness. A blister of Spanish flies applied to the part affected (after shaving off the hair), with a bath of strong spirits or vinegar, and a week's rest, will frequently suspend the lameness produced by the spavin for a time ; but a radical cure may not be expected.

ANOTHER.

Mr. Thornton :—During the year 1838, one of my carriage horses became badly spavined—so much so, as to render him useless for riding, being lame after using as well as before: I consulted the different farriers, and all agreed that it was incurable, and that the horse was useless. As such, I concluded I would try an experiment, and if it failed, I should only be where I was before with a useless horse. I accordingly had him tied in the usual way for castrating, thrown, and the legs well secured. Then with a common knife made an incision in the shape of a V, immediately over the knot, skinned it down, so as to present the knot ; I then took a firmer chisel, placing it where the spavin knot had joined the leg bone, and with a mallet cut the excrescence off as close as possible to the bone, then sewed up the skin, and in a few weeks the horse was well. It now has been three years, and the horse entirely restored. COLE.

ANOTHER.—*Editors of Cultivator.*—The following I have found would cure a bone spavin in its first stages, if properly applied. Add to two tablespoonsful of melted lard, one of cantharides, made fine or pulverized, and a lump of corrosive sublimate, pulverized, as large as a pea—all melted up together and applied once a day till used up, confining it to the callous. This quantity is for one leg, and may be relied on as a cure. It will make a sore, and the joint will be much weakened while applying the medicine, but no need of alarm; it will be all right when healed up. EDWARD D. WORBASSE.
Edon Farm, N. J. Aug. 15, 1843.

SWINEY.

Messrs. Editors.—I will give you such information or experience as I possess, concerning the swiney. I had a mare that became swineyed in the hip, occasioned by fighting with another horse. I was told the part affected never would fill up, unless by the operation of some medicine. I therefore bathed the part affected with saltpetre dissolved in water, and effected a complete cure. LANSINGVILLE.
Lansing, N. Y., Aug. 18, 1843.

THE GLANDERS.

From the Albany Cultivator.

Messrs. Editors.—Whilst writing, I will mention a fact for your veterinary department. More than thirty years since, the glanders, of the most virulent kind, was amongst the horses of the neighbourhood in which my father lived. Great numbers died off. His horse was taken, and under the belief that he also would die, my father commenced an experiment on him with a strong decoction of tobacco juice, given internally. In a short time the horse broke out all over his body in sores. These cured up in a month or so, and the horse was sound, soon fatted, and was, as I knew him afterwards, a sound and healthy animal. This was the only horse in all the neighbourhood that recovered. Some farmers in this vicinity, noted for fine sleek horses, give occasionally Scotch snuff to their horses. J. B. COOK.

BIG HEAD IN HORSES.

I have seen a number of horses that were afflicted with this disease. The first I attempted to cure was a horse about six years old, which a brother of mine obtained in the State of Tennessee. He had been subjected to the following treatment :—The duct that passes from the eye to the nose was laid bare, or an incision made in the large part of the nose, and the wound burned with a hot iron. This afforded a temporary relief. But the horse, about two years afterwards, became diseased; dwindled away, and lost, measurably, the use of parts. I had him thrown and tied; then run a hot iron through his head, inserting it into the lump on one side, and carrying it through the lump upon the other. The horse in a short time was well, and never after had any symptom of the disease. I have treated others in the same way, with equal success. I am no farrier, neither have I been able, by carefully examining the skull or head of several horses, to ascertain the cause of the disease. I know that it is a morbid enlargement of the bone of the head. It differs very much from the glanders. I think it certainly is not contagious. I have never heard of a mule that had it. J. A. M.

LAMPASS.

All young horses are subject to the lampass, and some suffer extremely before it is discovered.

It is a swelling or enlarging of the gums on the inside of the upper jaw; the growth is sometimes so large as to prevent a horse from eating with any comfort. The cure is simple, and after being performed, a horse will improve in his condition with great rapidity.

Take a hot iron, flat, sharp, and a little crooked at the end, burn the lampass out just below the level of the teeth, using great care to prevent the hot iron from bearing or resting on the teeth. After the operation is performed, the horse should be given a little bran or meal, with a small quantity of salt in it. Some farriers have recommended cutting for the lampass, which only gives momentary relief, and would require the same operation to be performed every three or four months; but when it is once burned out it never again makes it appearance.

HOOKS OR HAWS.

The hooks or haws in a horse is the growing of a horny substance upon the inner edge of the washer or caruncle of the eye, which may be found in the inner corner next to the nose. When this disease makes its appearance, the washer or caruncle is enlarged with great rapidity, and the ligament that runs along the edge of this membrane becomes extremely hard, or like a cartilage; and whenever it arises to this state, it draws, compresses, and causes great pain to the eyes, produces a tightness of the skin, a stiffness of the hind legs, and finally a general spasmodic affection throughout the whole system.

As the eyes are often inflamed, and sometimes diseased, without their having the hooks, for the purpose of ascertaining the fact, take hold of the bridle, and raise the horse's head as high as you can with convenience reach: if he is diseased with the hooks, the washer or caruncle of the eye, while his head is raised up, will cover at leest one half the surface of the eye-ball. When this is the case, take a common sized needle, with a strong thread, place on the horse's nose a twitch, to prevent his moving; then take in your thumb and finger the washer or caruncle of the eye, and pass the needle through it, about a quarter of an inch from the outer edge, and inside the horny substance; draw it gently with the needle and thread, until you have a fair chance of performing the operation; then with a sharp knife cut the piece out taken with the needle, which must not be larger than one fourth the size of a fourpence-halfpenny: wash the eyes for two or three mornings with salt and water, bathe his legs up to his belly in equal parts of warm vinegar, spirits, and oil, or fresh butter, and give a mash of one and a half gallons of bran or oats, one tablespoonful of flour of sulphur, one teaspoonful of saltpetre, and the cure will be performed, in all probability, in four or five days. Great care should be taken not to cut too large a piece from the caruncle, as it disfigures the eye, and sometimes produces blindness.

LOCKJAW.

The lockjaw being so fatal in its consequences, it is a fortunate circumstance it occurs so seldom among horses.

It commences with a difficulty in mastication; and

shortly after the jaws are so completely and immovably closed, that it is with much difficulty that medicine can be administered. The muscles of the neck appear to be much contracted, and the animal appears to suffer great pain.

The lockjaw is frequently brought on by trifling causes, such as cuts, wounding of nerves, tendons, &c. Generally speaking, the cure is uncertain; but it will chiefly depend on opium, the warm bath, and other anti-spasmodics. Sometimes the sudden application of cold water, in great quantities, has been serviceable; friction of turpentine, oil, or spirits, generally proves useful, as does a clyster made with two ounces of spirits of hartshorn, four ounces of oil of turpentine, and the yolk of three or four eggs, mixed with a quart of strong ale and gin or whiskey. It is a great object to promote urine, sweat, &c. Opium, camphor, and copious bleedings have been found, in some cases, very beneficial; and when they have failed, hartshorn, ether, opium, and brandy have been employed with some success; though the lockjaw is often a symptom of approaching dissolution, and frequently defies the power of any kind of medicine that can be employed.

GRAVEL IN THE HOOFS.

The gravel in the hoof is an incident that happens to horses in travelling, and is brought on by small stones or grit getting between the hoof and shoe, settling to the quick, and then inflaming and festering; it produces lameness, and causes a horse to undergo very excruciating pain. The first step necessary for a horse's relief is to have his shoes taken off and get the stones out. You may readily determine where they lie, by pressing the edge of the hoof with a pair of pincers, after all the gravel is removed, which may be known by a discontinuation of the blackness of the place. The wound caused by cutting for the gravel may be easily healed by melting together equal parts of beeswax, resin, fresh butter, or sweet oil, and pouring the mixture on the wound, warm as the animal can bear it without giving pain. Then warm a little tar or pitch, and pour a small quantity over the wound and its neighbouring parts to keep out the dust and defend the foot from any hard substance for a few days, by which time it will get well.

STONE OR GRAVEL IN THE BLADDER.

Fortunately the stone is a disease not very common among horses; but whenever it makes its appearance, unless some remedy is immediately employed, its consequences are to be much dreaded. It consists in small gravel or stones being lodged in the bladder, which prevent a free discharge of urine, and produce the most excruciating pain. The horse will linger and pine away until he can scarcely support the burden of life.

As the stone is a disease which has but seldom, if ever, struck the attention of farriers, I consider myself fortunate in being able to offer to the public a simple remedy, which has been employed with astonishing success by a gentleman in a neighbouring county. In one case, when the following remedy was used, three stones and a quantity of grit were discharged from the bladder.

Symptoms.—Frequent stretching, groaning, and many fruitless attempts to pass water, which will finally be discharged by a few drops at a time, with great apparent pain, a shrinking of the flesh, although the appetite is good, no fever, but a dull, sluggish, and sleepy appearance, wanting much in his usual spirits.

Remedy.—Take of marsh-mallows, water melon seed, and asparagus, of each two large handsful; boil them in three quarts of water to one quart, and add one teaspoonful of saltpetre, and give the whole as a drench, after being nicely strained.

Take of sweet oil or fresh butter one tablespoonful, grease his sheath, and draw out gently and grease his penis, also grease the large seam from the penis up near the anus; and with the hand, bearing a little, stroke the seam downward to the end of the penis, for ten minutes every hour, until the horse has a urinary discharge, which in all probability will take place in one or two hours after taking the drench. Should some blood be passed, it may be no cause of alarm, and will clearly prove there is gravel in the urinary passages. Repeat the dose in three hours, should the desired effect not be produced.

HIDE-BOUND.

A horse is said to be hide-bound when his skin will not slip under the pressure of the hand, but sticks as fast to the ribs as if it were glued.

Horses are sometimes hide-bound in consequence of feeling the effects of some violent disease, and it is often a bad symptom; but generally this tightness of the skin proceeds from poverty, cruel usage, and sometimes from worms.

The first thing necessary for performing a cure is to offer better treatment to the animal, giving him plenty of light food, such as bran, oats, &c., and a clean stable, with fresh litter. Then take from the neck vein half a gallon of blood. At night give a mash composed of one gallon of bran, scalded with sassafras tea, one tablespoonful of flour of sulphur, or powdered brimstone, and one teaspoonful of saltpetre, not permitting him to drink for six hours afterward. On the second day, at twelve o'clock, take of copperas two tablespoonsful, of warm sassafras tea one quart, saltpetre one teaspoonful. Mix and give them as a drench; have the horse well rubbed, and in a few days he will be entirely relieved.

YELLOW WATER.

The yellow water is very common in the western country among horses; and being infectious, is sometimes brought into this State by drove horses. It is extremely fatal in its consequences, unless some remedy is employed shortly after it makes its appearance. For the benefit of the public, I consider myself fortunate to be able to recommend such medicines for its cure as have been fairly tried by a gentleman of Brunswick, and proved effectual.

Symptoms of yellow water —The characteristics of this disease are a dusky yellowne s of the eyes, lips, and bars of the mouth; a dull, sluggish appearance, a loss of appetite, the excrement hard, dry, yellow, and sometimes of a pale or light green; the urine uncommonly dark, of a dirty brown colour, and when discharged a length of time has the appearance of blood.

Remedy.—Take of asafœtida one ounce; camphorated spirits, four tablespoonsful; warm water, one pint; mix and give them as a drench, for three or four mornings successively: take of bran, one and a half gallons; flour of sulphur, one tablespoonful;

antimony, twenty grains; mix them well together, and with a strong decoction of sassafras, scald the bran, forming a mash, which must be given three nights in the week, not permitting the horse to get wet, or drink water, except it is milk-warm; his stable should be a comfortable one, and he should have a clean bed of straw placed under him. Bleed twice in the neck vein, taking half a gallon of blood at each bleeding, within the week; let his exercise be regular and moderate, and by the expiration of nine or ten days, the cure, in all probability, will be performed.

REMEDY FOR THE BOTTS.

Some six years since, I purchased a very fine horse, which had the appearance of labouring under some disease. I commenced a course of treatment which I thought would relieve him, and which I had pursued in the treatment of some other horses which had the appearance of being diseased in a similar manner to the above mentioned horse, with decided relief; but in this case all my remedies failed of their desired effect.

I was induced to try the use of lime in the treatment of his case, as I was confident he was filled with grubs or botts, as he had discharged several. I commenced by giving him a tablespoonful of slacked lime three times per week, in bread mashes. After pursuing this course near two weeks, the botts began to pass off in quantities, varying from ten to twenty, which he would expel during the night from his intestines. In the meantime his appetite began to improve, and in six weeks he was one of the finest looking geldings I ever saw. From that day to this I have kept up the use of lime among my horses with decided benefit.

As an evidence of its good effects, I have not lost a horse since I began to use it. A large number of the botts which he would expel from his intestines had the appearance of being dead. I was induced from this fact to put some of them in a strong solution of lime water, as I had frequently put them in spirits of turpentine, without producing any effect on them; but all those that I put into lime were perfectly dead in eight-and-forty hours.

Lime is a certain preventive in keeping cattle from taking the murrain. As an evidence of this fact I have used it among my cattle three times per week, mixed with salt, for three or four years. In that time I have not lost a single cow, or steer, or ox, by this disease; in the mean time, some of my neighbours have lost nearly all the cattle they owned.

I will give you a stronger case than the one above mentioned:—One of my neighbours, who lost all his cattle, had a neighbour living within two hundred yards of him, who had several cattle which ran daily with those that died, and his cattle all escaped. He informed me he had made it an invariable rule to give his cattle salt and lime every morning. I have no doubt it is a sure and infallible remedy for botts in horses, and a preventive of murrain among cattle.

J. W. J.

Red House, N. C., Nov. 16, 1839.

ANOTHER.—On no subject has a greater number of receipts been published. We here record one, which comes to us in an Ohio Paper, the Marietta Farmer. It has the recommendation of being plain and brief, and of being sanctioned by the name of the writer.

To make botts let go their hold, give the horse a

quantity of molasses or dissolved sugar, with a quart of sweet milk; in thirty minutes you will find the horse at ease. Then pulverize an eighth of a pound of alum, dissolved in a quart of warm water, and drench your horse. After two hours, or less, give the horse one pound of salts, and you will find the botts in the dung. I have never failed. I think this is, after all the speculations and cures that I have seen, the only thing that will, to a certainty, remove the botts. The molasses and sweet milk will cause the botts to let go, and prey upon the sweetening. The alum contracts them, and the salts pass them off.

J. C. WALTER.

ANOTHER,—by Baron Steuben's farrier, who came to this country with him during the revolutionary war, in the year 1778.—He was called a man of great skill and celebrity in his profession. The ingredients are simple, and too mild to produce any injurious effects on the animal to which they may be administered. They consist of new milk, honey or molasses, common salt and water, and linseed oil. The manner of preparing and administering is as follows: As soon as the disease (the symptoms of which are unerring) is ascertained, drench the horse, fasting if possible, with a quart of fresh milk saturated with honey, molasses, or sugar; to be preferred in the order stated. Leave him at rest for two hours; at the expiration of which, having previously prepared some strong brine, by boiling as much common salt as can be dissolved in it, drench him as before with a pint of it when cool. After a similar period of two hours, give him half a pint of linseed oil, and the remedy is complete.

TO KILL LICE ON HORSES, COWS AND HOGS.

From the Central New York Farmer.

Take the water in which potatoes have been boiled, rub it all over the skin. The lice will be dead within two hours, and never will multiply again. I have used ten kinds of the strongest poison to kill lice, all with effect, but none so perfect as this. M. T.

DISTEMPER IN CATTLE

May be cured by boiling the common poke-root to a strong decoction, and administering a quart of it three times a day.

DISEASES AND TREATMENT OF CATTLE.

Imported into the South, by Col. W. Hampton,

All cattle imported from England, the North and West, are very liable to be attacked with a fatal disease, which I take to be an inflammation of the brain.

Young cattle, from eight months to one year old, are less subject to it than those more advanced in life. If they survive the summer and autumn, I consider them safe, although great care should be taken of them the second season. They should be brought into the State as early in the fall as possible, kept in good growing condition through the winter, and in the spring be removed to a high healthy position, have easy access to pure water, and their pasture as much shaded as the nature of the ground will admit. In August and September, they should be kept in a cool stable during the heat of the day, and at night also, the dew at that season being almost as injurious as the intense heat of the sun.

With these precautions, I think more than half would escape the disease, the first indication of which is usually a languid appearance of the animal, followed by the loss of appetite, short quick breathing, with more or less fever, and not unfrequently accompanied by a cough.

I have hitherto considered this disease, when once established, incurable. I have recently learned, however, that by sawing off the horns, close to the head, nine out of ten would recover. They may be bled copiously, which relieves the dullness about the eyes. After the bleeding is stopped, bind cloths plastered with tar, around the stump, as a protection against flies.

TO KILL LICE ON CATTLE.

We have been informed by a gentleman who has for many years kept a large stock of cattle, that fine dry sand scattered on the back, neck, and sides of the animals, is an effectual remedy against these vermin. He collects dry sand, and puts it in a box or tub in the barn, and occasionally applies it during the winter, by sifting or strewing it over the body of each creature with complete success in ridding it of its troublesome guests.

ANOTHER.—Make a strong sassafras tea, or red pepper tea, or a mixture of both is preferable, with a reasonable portion of lard, and rub or wash the animal with it every two or three days. It will kill the lice and destroy the nits as fast as they hatch, and, by a few washings, the animal will soon be rid of the lice. It is a sure and safe remedy.

TO DESTROY VERMIN ON CATTLE.

A strong decoction of tobacco, washed over a beast infected with vermin, will generally drive them away. It sometimes will make the beast very sick for a short time. But a better remedy, is to mix plenty of strong Scotch snuff in train oil, and rub the back and neck of the creature with it, which will effectually kill or drive away all vermin from a quadruped.

TO DESTROY VERMIN ON CATTLE AND TO CURE THE MANGE.

Put into an earthen vessel four ounces of flour of sulphur, and a pound weight of nut oil; place the vessel upon a moderate fire, and stir the mixture with a piece of wood, until part of the flour of sulphur is dissolved, and the oil has acquired a reddish-brown colour; then remove it from off the fire; and before it is entirely cold, add four ounces of essence of turpentine; then stir it again, until it is incorporated. This preparation is neither expensive nor complicated; and when used, is merely put upon the parts infected with a feather.

HORN DISTEMPER, OR HORN AIL.

Is a disorder incident to horned cattle, by which the internal substance of the horn (commonly called the pith, which is the spongy part of the bone), wastes away, &c. This disorder may be known by a dullness in the countenance, a sluggish motion, want of appetite, a desire to lie down frequently, shaking the head, and appearing dizzy, &c. To be sure of this disease, take a small gimlet and perforate the horn two or three inches above the head: if it is hollow, and no blood follows, it is the hollow horn. This distemper is generally brought on by poverty, &c.

Bore each horn at the upper and lower side, that the drain may have vent, and administer at least two or three doses of salts, or some gentle purgative;

inject into the horn strong vinegar. This will cleanse the horn, and effect a cure. Sawing off the horn is sometimes performed, but the above receipt is preferable.

HOOF-AIL.
From the Cultivator.

Messrs. Editors.—Perceiving in your last number, an inquiry respecting the hoof-ail in cattle, I am happy to have it in my power to communicate one which never fails in effecting a cure in two or three days. Blue vitriol finely pulverized, and applied to the diseased part of the hoof, once a day for two or three days, is all that is necessary. In the case of a cow of mine, one application was sufficient; and, I presume, would generally answer the purpose. The disease here is called by some of our farmers, "fouls," and by others hoof-ail. If the case alluded to by your correspondent is the same disease, you can depend on my remedy. E. H. Hubbarb.

Middletown, Ct., 1840.

Another.—This disease is generally brought on by driving cattle on hard or muddy roads. The first symptom is lameness. When this is noticed, the foot on examination will be found to be in some degree inflamed and swollen. Wash the foot in pickle as strong as you can make it. This has frequently proved effectual, but if it does not, an ointment made of corrosive sublimate and hog's lard, rubbed in the slit between the hoofs, is a good remedy; if it be neglected, the parts below the hoof will become dry and horny, in which case the hard part must be cut out, and the wounded flesh cured with healing ointment.

ON THE DISEASE COMMONLY CALLED THE HOLLOW HORN.

There is perhaps no disease in this climate from

which our neat cattle have suffered so much as that commonly called the hollow horn, and unfortunately, few persons have thought it necessary to give any attention to it or its cure, for we find but little said in any agricultural work relative to its treatment.

The name appears to me to be badly applied, as the horn alone is not the seat of the disease: it pervades the whole system, and cattle without horns are quite as subject to it as those with them—having often seen those without horns have it.

The hollowness of the horn proceeds from the violence of the fever throughout the system. I have known cattle feeding in the stall to be attacked with it, as well as those in a poor condition, and, no doubt, those in bad plight are more liable to its attack, their systems not being in a state to resist any disease. It occurs, too, at all seasons of the year, but more particularly in the spring.

The animal attacked with it looks rough, stares much in its coat, and falls off very fast in flesh, its food having but little effect in nourishing it; the eyes look very hollow and dead, and run with a yellow matter, which collects in the corners, and around them. Many persons rely upon the feel of the horn as the best indication of the disease, but this I think very uncertain: in some cases, it is at the root cold to the feel, while in others very hot. A very small gimblet will, however, remove all doubts, and the mark on the horn not be visible after a few days. If the disease does exist, the horn will be found without pith, and little or no blood will follow the boring; whereas, if the disease does not exist, you will find blood immediately upon entering the horn. The gimblet used for boring should be well washed and greased after boring; for if it is not, and should be used to try the horns of animals not actually infected with the disease, it will most generally give it to them. It is a disease that is highly inflammatory and infectious, and the animal having it ought to be removed from the herd until well.

The following mode of treatment I have found very successful, and the beast is soon restored to a thriving state. As soon as I discover an animal affected with the hollow horn, I bleed it from the neck (in the same vein in which a horse is bled), from two to six or seven quarts, according to its age, size, and condition, and administer three quarters to one pound and a half of glauber salts; with a middle-sized gimblet open the horns through and through, marking the holes, so that they be perpendicular in the usual position the animal carries its head, so that the pus formed may have a free discharge as soon as the horns are opened; put through the hole into each about a tablespoonful of strong vinegar, in which some salt and black pepper, ground, has been put. The day following, the horns must be again opened, and cleansed from the pus, which generally is now formed, and about half a teaspoonful of spirits of turpentine put into each horn; and a little on the poll of the animal daily, during the continuance of the disease. One bleeding is generally sufficient, but I have known cases in which it was necessary to repeat it three times, as also the salts. The food during the continuance of the disease is important—corn in every shape is bad—potatoes are of great use (with a small quantity of brewer's grains if it be had); and the animal ought to have from one to two and a half pecks daily, with hay in the winter, and grass if in the summer. Potatoes have a wonderful effect on the animal, as soon as the bowels are well cleansed; the importance of which any person will be convinced of who observes the discharge of the animal. In some obstinate cases, I have given daily from a half to one ounce of nitre sprinkled with potatoes. It is important the first bleeding, to take as much blood as the animal will bear, as the fever is more easily checked by one large bleeding than two small ones, and the animal better able to bear it. In many cases the bleeding and salts have been sufficient without opening the horns, and when taken in the early stage will generally be found to answer; but the boring certainly assists in forming anew the internal part of the horn, and as soon as it commences forming, the holes in the horn should be allowed to close. An animal having the hollow horn should be sheltered from the inclemency of the weather, during its continuance. No age appears exempt from its attacks. I have seen it in a yearling, as well as at all subsequent ages.

I am induced to offer this mode of treatment to your subscribers, having never in any instance failed of restoring the animal: whereas, before this mode of treatment was adopted, I annually lost several. The fleam for bleeding cattle should be rather deeper than that used for a horse, the vein in the neck not lying so near the surface: the orifice is closed with a pin, in the same way as in bleeding a horse.

HOW TO RELIEVE CHOKED CATTLE.

It will be recollected by the constant readers of the Telegraph, that some months since, John Conant, of this village, published an article in the Telegraph, addressed to Farmers, making known a method for relieving cattle choked with potatoes, or other substances. The object of this paragraph is to call attention to the subject again, and to add my own testimony in favor of the remedy.

A few mornings since one of my cows was choked with a potatoe. Living but a short distance from my friend Conant, I sent for his assistance, as I had never witnessed the operation. He came with a quantity of gunpowder, took about as much as would be necessary to charge a common fowling-piece two or three times, enclosed it in paper, somewhat after the manner of preparing a cartridge, and while I held the cow's head up, he, with his hand, thrust the preparation down her throat as far as convenient. I held her head up a moment, until she had broken and swallowed the charge, which soon produced heaving; but the first trial did not succeed. After waiting a few minutes we repeated the process, which succeeded admirably, and the poor, distressed animal was relieved at once; she raised the potatoe, chewed, and swallowed it.—*Vermont Telegraph.*

ANOTHER.—Mr. Josiah D. Smith, of the county of Henrico, desires us to say to his brother farmers, that after an ineffectual resort to the usual remedies, he relieved a choked ox, a few days since, by holding up his head, and pouring into his mouth a strong solution of soap in water. The relief was instantaneous, the turnip with which he was choked passing down immediately into the stomach.

HOVEN CATTLE.

One of my cows, a very valuable animal of the common breed, lately became bloated or "hoven," in consequence of getting into the barn-floor through a door which was carelessly left open, and eating her fill of potatoes. She was swelled up as tight as the skin could hold, in about twelve or fifteen hours after eating them. Upon discovering the painful and dangerous situation of the cow, I immediately sent for a neighbour who had frequently relieved hoven cattle by plunging a knife into the paunch, and thus affording an exit for the confined air. This was done first with a pen-knife, then with a Spanish dirk-knife, without the desired effect, no air escaping through the puncture. Being anxious to relieve the suffering animal, it occured to me that what would be beneficial in the human being, under similar circumstances, or in Tympanites intestinalis, might possibly give relief. I lost no time until I had a decoction of anise and fennel-seed, prepared by boiling for a few minutes a handful composed of equal quantities of the two, in a pint of water. This I added to one pound of hog's lard, and bridling the cow, raised her head by pulling the reins over the top-rail of a fence, and gave it to her in the usual way. She appeared to be sinking so fast now, that we drove her out to a field to die. When there, she soon laid down, very much exhausted, and panting laboriously, seemed to be rapidly approaching the end of her sufferings. I now concluded to try another dose of the carminative and lard, having observed that she frequently eructated, since giving the first dose; we accordingly had another prepared, in all respects like the first. This we had no difficulty in getting down, as she lay, without the bridle. Shortly after the exhibition of this dose, the air began to roll in large and frequently repeated volumes, up the gullet—this effect of the medicine continuing at short intervals—in half an hour the cow was quite relieved, and walking about. The effect of this simple remedy was indeed most admirable, and deserves to be known by every person owning a cow. One of my neighbors has since experienced the good effects of it in the case of a cow that had become hoven in consequence of eating corn, and corn fodder in the shock. It may not be amiss to mention that the lard in the above prescription, was recommended, in the first place as a purgative, and therefore became part of the drench. Tar was put upon the puncture, and it healed kindly. R. NEBINGER.

Lewisburg, Pa., October 20, 1841.

REMEDY FOR SWELLINGS, OR SNARLED BAGS IN COWS.

Cows, soon after calving, are subject to have swellings or knots in their udders; this is more particularly the case with heifers with their first calves. It sometimes proceeds from colds contracted prior to calving; at others, from the inability of the calf to extract all the milk, which throws the cow into a feverish condition, and the formation of indurated surfaces consequently follows. Should fever accompany these lumps, a little cooling medicine will be proper, as a solution of half a pound of Epsom salts in a drench, to be followed with good nourishing messes, say one peck of bran, and half a pound of flaxseed meal, to be first boiled, and given warm, morning and night, for a few days. To reduce the swelling in the udder, the following receipt will be found excellent:

Take a handful of rue, and the same quantity of wormseed; bruise them both well, and put them into a skillet or other vessel, with a pound of unsalted butter, fresh from the churn; simmer the whole well over a slow fire for an hour; then strain the mixture through a sieve or linen cloth, and you have the best ointment that can be applied. Let the inflamed and hardened part be gently anointed three times a day with the hand, and in a few days the cure will be effected, if this remedy is applied in time.

Care should always be taken before the calf is turned to the cow, for several days after she has calved, to let the dairy woman draw off a portion of the milk; by so doing you are sure the calf will extract the rest: by thus emptying the cow's udders you will prevent the ill consequences which ensue where a part of the milk is left in the bag to produce fever and snarls.

A CURE FOR MURRAIN.

From the Genesee Farmer.

MESSRS. EDITORS.—I have seen several inquiries respecting the murrain in cattle, and being in possession of a receipt which, in nine cases out of ten, has proved successful in curing the same, I herewith send it to you, in hopes that if you give it publicity, it may be of some benefit to those who are yearly losing many of their cattle.

Receipt.—Give one and a half ounces pearlash, dissolved in two quarts of iron-water (from a blacksmith's trough). If not better in five hours, give half an ounce more in one quart of water. The water should be warm. Give no drink but warm water, for two days. Give warm mash to eat.

THOMAS FORSYTH.

Chatham, Canada, April 10, 1843.

CURE FOR THE BLOODY MURRAIN.

Mr. Joseph Priestman communicated to the Genesee Farmer the following cure for this fatal disease:

Take a piece of poke-root, as large as a man's fist, say half a pound in weight, cut it fine, add two quarts of water, boil it down to one quart. This quantity must be given once a day, for two or three days, to a cow or bull, when the cure will have been effected.

CURE FOR MURRAIN AND YELLOW WATER IN CATTLE.

For Murrain.—Glauber salts, one pound; nitre and cream of tartar in powder, each one ounce; ginger pulverized, two ounces; treacle or molasses, four teaspoonsful; mix for a dose. If it does not succeed in twenty-four hours, add strained turpentine, four ounces; Armenian bale bayberries, and red saunders in powder, of each two ounces; mix in a mortar, and beat it into a proper consistence for the bale or ball.

Taken from the Notes of Captain George D. Porter, of the British Navy, in 1829,—who, until he tried this, was losing every hoof he had, in Tyrone county, north of Ireland, but lost none afterwards. My father has a great number of mountainous farms there; and ascribed the hale and healthy condition of his cattle very much to constant bleeding, which the herds practised, for eating the same. For yellow water, or blood with urine, arising from bad or sanded hay,—1. Drench with Barbadoes aloes, half an ounce; common salt, four ounces: ginger, one drachm; water, one quart; anodyne carminative tincture, two ounces; or substitute for the latter one tablespoonful of opium. 2. Drench with Epsom salts, six or eight ounces; water, one pint; castor oil, eight ounces; cream or half made butter, with the whey, as a substitute for the oil, and four ounces of common salt substitute for the Epsom salts. A wine-glass of brandy or gin will do for the laudanum or tincture.

SALT FOR CATTLE.

Let it be remembered, that salt, when given to animals, enables the farmer to increase his live stock, and keep them in health : hence it ought freely to be given to sheep, and cattle of every description ; but, to imitate nature, it should be previously dissolved, and then mixed with pure, fine clay, in a mass, which is to be placed under a shelter, so that the animals may lap it at pleasure.

A CURE FOR SCOURS IN CALVES.

Take a tablespoonful of finely powdered chalk, and a like quantity of ground ginger, put it in a bowl, pour boiling new milk on it, say half a pint ; stir it well, and then give this dose about milk warm night and morning to the calf, and in nine cases out of ten two doses will be sufficient.

Farmer and Gardner.

DISEASES OF CALVES.

The diseases of calves are principally confined to a species of convulsions which now and then attacks them, and which sometimes arises from worms, and at others from cold. When the first cause operates, it is relieved by giving a mild aloetic purge, or in default of that, a mild dose of oil of turpentine, half an ounce night and morning. In the second, wrap up the animal warm, and drench with ale and laudanum a drachm. Calves are also subject to diarrhœa, or scouring, which will readily yield to the usual medicines.

CURE FOR POISONED SHEEP.

In the spring of the year sheep and lambs are very apt to eat the green leaves of the low laurel, camp-kill, as it is sometimes called. This brings on a retching or vomiting of a greenish fluid, which the sheep again swallow down. The animal begins to swell and becomes stupid, refuses to eat or drink, and finally dies. As soon as a sheep is discovered to be sick, and throw up the fluid above mentioned, fix a gag in its mouth by taking a short stick, or a corn cob, tying a string at each end, put it into the mouth, and passing the string up over the head of the sheep so as to keep the gag in, and the mouth open. This prevents them from swallowing. A dose of weak ammonia is very good. Roasted onions put under the fore legs are also beneficial. A communication by Mr. Newman, of Worcester, Mass., in the last number of the New England Farmer, recommends a strong decoction of the bruised twigs of white ash, given in doses of two spoonsful to a sheep, especially if administered within the last twenty-four hours after the sheep has eaten the poison.

DISEASES OF SHEEP.
From the Silk Culturist.

The great losses which wool-growers frequently sustain in consequence of the sickness and death of large numbers of their flocks, have induced us to compile from a rare and valuable English work a synopsis of the diseases to which sheep are liable, together with the symptoms by which they are known, and the treatment by which they are remedied. The causes of the disease are in some cases assigned, and it is believed if they are carefully avoided, and the remedies promptly and faithfully applied, the losses from disease and death will in a great degree be prevented, and the profits arising from their fleeces and young be materially increased. As the remedies are simple, and the ingredients composing the prescriptions within the reach of every farmer, it is to be hoped that every wool-grower who has the misfortune to have a diseased flock will give them a thorough trial.

Fever.—Fever in sheep is an inflamed state of the blood, disordering the eye and mouth, and affecting the whole body, though not visibly. When any of the symptoms of a fever appear, the feet of the sheep should be examined, and if found to be hot, there is no doubt of the character of the disease: other diseases will produce an inflammation of the eyes and mouth, but hot feet are an infallible symptom of fever. This disease is often fatal in itself, and frequently induces others which are equally so. The cause is generally a cold. When only two or three of the flock are affected by it, the case is less desperate; but when many are attacked with it, it is more fatal. The remedy is to keep the sheep in warmer and more sheltered places; bleed and give the following medicine :—

Heat a quart of ale, and dissolve in it an ounce of nithritate, add half an ounce of Virginia snake-root, and one drachm cochineal in powder. This quantity serves for four doses, and one of them is to be given morning and evening. If the sheep is bound in its body, an ounce of sanative electuary is to be mixed with each dose; but if looser than ordinary, it ought not to be checked, as it will contribute to the cause.

Purging.—Leave nature to her course when a purging comes on with a fever; but when the fever is abated, it should be stopped; and the same remedy that answers for this purpose may be adopted for such purgings as come on of themselves. Boil a quarter of a pound of raspings of logwood in two quarts of water till but a quart is left, and when it is nearly boiled down, put in a stick of cinnamon, strain it off, and give the sheep a quarter of a pint, four times a day till the purging ceases. If this does not produce the desired result, the following addition will render it sure of success :—To every dose, add a quarter of an ounce of diascordium without honey, and ten grains of Japan earth powdered, and give the doses only morning and evening.

Tag.—The tag is an external disease, owing to the complaint last named. It is a distemper of the tail, beginning with filth and foulness, and ending in ulceration. The tag is situated in the inner part of the tail; it consists of scabs and sores, very painful and wasting to the animal, and is owing to the fouling of this part by purging; that tag is worst which follows a fever, because the inflamed state of the blood tends to increase the disorder, and when it begins during the continuance of the disease, the matter of the fever may chance to settle it there. Two things are to be done; the first is to stop the purging, and the other to clean the tail. The last mentioned remedy, either in its weaker or stronger form, is to be used to stop the purging, and the tail being clipped, and the sore part laid bare, first wash it with milk and water, blood-warm, and then with lime water; after this turn the sheep into a clean dry pasture. Two days after look at it again, and if not well, repeat the washing, and anoint it with grease and tar mixed together. Twice doing of this is generally sufficient to complete the cure.

Disease of the lungs.—Sheep are subject to be

diseased in the lungs, which is easily perceived by their breathing or by their coughing. Nothing requires a more speedy remedy, for they grow incurable when it is neglected a short time, and die as men with a consumption. Change of their pasture is essential to the cure ; without it, no remedy is effectual. It is owing to cold, and generally attacks sheep that have been kept on low grounds in wet weather. When any of the flock exhibit symptoms of diseased lungs, drive them into an enclosed pasture where there is short grass and a gravelly soil, and where there is spring or other running water; bruise a basketful of the leaves of colts-foot, and press out the juice ; bruise a quantity of plantain leaves and roots together, and press out the juice; mix these, and bruise as much garlic as will yield about a fourth part as much juice as one of the others ; mix all together, and add to them a pound of honey, an ounce of anise-seed, and an ounce and a half of elecampane ; give a quarter of a pint of this warm once in a day, to every sheep that is affected, and it will, by degrees, make a perfect cure.

Jaundice.—Sheep are more subject than any other animals to obstructions of the liver. When this is the case, it is seen in a yellowness of the eyes, and a tint of the same kind in the skin. Farmers, in some places, call this the choler, or, in their language, the colour. When sheep are attacked with jaundice they should be put into an open pasture, and kept in moderate motion, but not fatigued. Boil in four gallons of water, two pounds of fennel roots, the same quantity of parsley roots, and twice as much roots of cough grass, all cut small. When the water is very strong of them, and there is about half the quantity left, strain it off by pressing it hard; bruise as much great celandine as will yield three pints of juice; add this to the liquor, and put in three drachms of salt of steel; mix all together, and every day beat as much of it as will serve to give every sheep that is ill a gill and a half for a dose. This, with the fore-mentioned directions, rarely fails of a cure.

Stoppage in the throat.—Sheep affected with stoppage in the throat wheeze and breathe with difficulty. It is commonly occasioned by bad pasturage and colds. The remedy is to put them on higher ground; keep them warm, and give them the following medicine:—Bruise a good quantity of pennyroyal, and squeeze out the juice; put to a quart of it a pound of honey and half a pint of sharp vinegar; give half a pint of this, blood-warm, every night.

Sturdiness.—This is a giddiness in the head. It is owing, principally, to rich feeding. The remedy is as follows: Bleed profusely, and give the following medicine: bruise some roots of wild valerian, squeeze out the juice, heat it, and give a quarter of a pint: repeat the dose every four hours. When the sheep is recovered, turn it upon the common, or into some barren, hilly pasture. It will be kept from relapses by having but little food, and that perfectly wholesome. If the disease returns, it is commonly fatal.

Wood evil.—This disease is a kind of cramp; it seizes the legs, and will often attack a whole flock at once. Cold and wet are the cause; lying under the drip of trees in rainy seasons has often occasioned it, and hence its name. In order to effect a cure, the sheep must be removed to a dry pasture, and there proper remedies may take effect. The following medicine is recommended:—Boil in a large quantity of ale, as much cinquefoil, and hedge mustard, as can be well stirred into it. When the liquor is very strong strain it off, and add a pint of juice of valerian root to every gallon; give half a pint of this morning and evening; boil in vinegar a large quantity of the leaves of hedge mustard, and with the liquor hot rub the legs.

Staggers.—Sheep, as well as horses, are sometimes afflicted with the staggers. It is occasioned by improper food. Oak leaves and buds are particularly prejudicial. They bind the bowels, and staggers frequently follow. The symptoms are the same as in sturdiness, but more violent, and there is generally a trembling at the same time in all the limbs. To cure this disorder, dissolve half an ounce of asafœtida in two quarts of water; give a quarter of a pint, warm, every three hours. It commonly opens the bowels at the same time that it takes immediate effect on the nervous system, and thus performs a cure. When the sheep are recovered, let them be kept out of the way of a return to the same food, and they will be in no danger of a relapse.

Another.—Half a pint of hog's lard melted and poured down a sheep will cure the blind staggers in ten minutes.

Scab.—This is a disorder to which sheep are very liable. When they are kept in dry wholesome pastures they are but seldom afflicted with the scab; but when they are on low wet grounds, or get under the drippings of trees in bad seasons, they are frequently affected by it in the severest manner. The symptoms are scurvy skins, which in a little time rise to scabs; the wool grows loose, and the sheep pine and become lean. If they are attacked in a season when they can be sheared, it should be immediately done, as nothing is so sure to effect a cure. If the season will not admit of shearing, they must be washed with soap-suds, made very strong, and used warm with a piece of flannel or a brush. After this, they must be let loose into a clean pasture, and driven up again as soon as well dried, and the sore parts of the skin must be well wetted with lime-water. The scurvy part of the skin must be regarded; and the doing this three times at intervals of two days will generally effect a cure. But if it fail, the parts that have been thus washed and cleansed must be anointed with a mixture of equal parts of tar and grease, and they will soon be perfectly well. No inward medicines are required, for the complaint is only of the skin.

Another.—Mr. Wheeler also writes us, that his flock were so much afflicted with scab that he lost one hundred, and his fleeces were diminished eleven cents per pound in consequence of the diseased state of the animals. He cured them of disease, and restored his flock to fine condition, in which they still remain, by the following :—He boiled eight pounds of tobacco in eight pailsful of water, down to five pailsful; to this he added five pailsful of weak ley from wood ashes, one barrel of soft soap, and some soft water. Filling in part a half hogshead with the liquid, he dipped into it three hundred and fifty sheep, liquid being added as required; the sheep, as fast as they were dipped, were placed in another tub, and the liquid pressed out of the fleece with the hands. The wash cleanses the skin from all scurf, kills the lice and ticks, promotes perspiration, and greatly facilitates the growth of the fleece and health of the animal. There is no doubt of the utility of any application that destroys the lice and ticks, and fits the skin, by thoroughly cleansing it, to perform its all-important functions.

Red Water.—This is an inflammation of the skin that often raises it into blisters, in which is contained a sharp humour, thin, watery and coloured with blood. Nothing should be done to strike it in, but the cure must be effected by correcting the bad state of the blood. Sheep afflicted with it should be separated from the flock, otherwise it will be apt to spread through the whole. They should also be put into a pasture where the grass is sweet, and where they can have access to good water. Mix half an ounce of sulphur with an ounce of honey; work it well together, and then divide it into two parts; dissolve one of these in half a pint of juice of nettles, and give it every day for a fortnight. Slit the blisters when they are full of this watery humour, and having let the matter out, wet the place with juice of wormwood; after four days of this course, bleed them, and then continue the same method till they are well.

Foot Worm.—Sheep are liable to breed worms between their feet, principally, however, when they are kept in wet pastures. It is very painful to them, and will make them pine away. It is perceived by their frequently holding up one foot, and by setting it tenderly down. Let the foot be washed clean, particularly between the toes, and there will be found a little lump, like a tuft of hair; this is the head of the wound. It is to be taken out with care, for it is of a tender substance, and if it be broken in the foot it will occasion inflammation. The best method is to open the flesh on each side of it, and then, by means of a pair of nippers, to take it out. Dress the wound with tar and grease, melted together in equal quantities, and turn the sheep loose. It is better to put them into a fresh pasture; for, if the same disorder returns, it is generally worse.

Wildfire.—This is a violent inflammation, not unlike St. Anthony's fire, upon the skin in different places, and generally affects the whole flock. Our forefathers used to bury the sheep alive, with its feet upward, at the door of the fold, superstitiously believing that it acted as a spell to drive away the disease. The following, however, is a more rational and modern method of cure. Separate such as are affected with the disease from the flock, bleed, and prepare the following external remedy: Bruise the leaves of wild chervil, and add to them as much lime water as will make the whole very soft; when it is beaten up together, add as much powder of fenugreek seed as will reduce it to pap; then put it into a pan, and set it in a cool place; rub the inflamed part carefully with this every evening, and make as much lie on as can be kept there; it will take effect during the time of rest, and is to be repeated as long as there is occasion.

Disorders of the eyes.—Sheep are often affected with colds falling upon their eyes, and almost blinding them; and, at other times, the same accident without any visible cause. The remedy in either case is the same. Press out the juice of great celandine, and drop a quantity of it into the eyes, night and morning.

Dropsy.—Sheep are often swelled with water in their bellies; and this, if not regarded in time, is certain death. There are two parts in which it is lodged; the one is between the outward flesh and the rind, the other within the rind. The first is easily cured ; for the other, nothing can be done. The method in the first case is, by a coarse kind of tapping. An opening is to be made in the flesh, and a quill thrust in. This will give the water a free passage out, and the wound heals of itself. But when the sheep is emaciated, nature will not have strength to heal it; and the sheep must be examined daily, and the wound dressed with tar and grease. It must also be put into a fresh, dry, and wholesome pasture, and then disposed of as soon as recruited; for this is a disorder that never fails to return upon any mismanagement in keeping.

The rot.—This is the most destructive disease to which sheep are subject. Like the murrain, it is contagious, and generally spreads through the whole flock, and often over the neighbouring country. Flocks that are fed upon open commons are more subject to it than such as have shelter and are taken care of at night. It frequently prevails in cold seasons, and when drizzling rains come on soon after shearing. Want of food will also occasion this disease, as will likewise the eating of such grass as is full of unwholesome plants. These are among the causes of this fatal distemper; but the worst and most common is infection. Keep sheep out of the way of these causes of the rot, and the same care will preserve them from most other disorders to which they are liable; damp grounds are always dangerous, and especially in wet seasons. When a sheep is infected with the rot, the white of the eyes looks dull, and they have a faint aspect; the animal is feeble, and his skin foul; the wool comes off in handsful at the least touch, and the gums look pale and the teeth foul; he will also be dull, and listless in motion, and heavy, as if his legs were not able to carry him. Many are generally affected at a time, and the first care must be to remove them from the sound ones, and put them in a close fold. They must have but little water, and their food must be hay and oats. Bleeding is destructive in the rot. The fact that sheep fed in salt marshes never have the rot, suggested salt as a remedy. It is a good preventive, and an infallible cure. Though the farmer cannot rely upon it, yet, among other remedies, it is highly useful. The following remedies and treatment have often effected cures: Bruise an ounce of the grains of paradise, and four ounces of juniper berries, dried; add to these four pounds of bay salt, and half a pound of loaf sugar; grind them well together, and sprinkle some of this upon the hay and oats that are given the sheep. Let this be continued three days, and look, from time to time, to the eyes, and examine every other way to see whether they mend or grow worse. If there be signs of amendment, let the same course be continued; if not, the following must be used: Steep four pounds of antimony in two gallons of ale, for a week; then give the sheep this every night and morning, a quarter of a pint at a time. Boil a pound of the roots of avens, and two pounds of the roots of masterwort in two gallons of water, till there are not more than six quarts remaining; strain this off and press it hard; then pour a pint of it into a pailful of water that is to be given to the sheep for their drink. By these means, carefully managed, and under a good regulation in cleanness, dryness, and warmth, the rot will often be cured. This is all that can be promised; for there are times when the disease is so rooted, and when the temperature of the air so favours it, that nothing will get the better of it. If the sheep have a distaste to the food, because of the salt and other ingredients mixed among it, they must be omitted for two or three feedings, and then given in less quantity.

Stretches.—This is the name given by a contributor to a late number of the Cultivator, to a disease which has been noticed among sheep, but which has hitherto been nameless. Many of the cases which had fallen under the notice of the writer in that Journal had proved fatal in from two to eight days after the attack; and, where not fatal, were seriously injurious to their general health, and consequently to the quantity and quality of the wool. We have noticed the complaint referred to, having within a year or two had three or four sheep thus attacked, though in no case has it proved fatal in our flock. It occurs only in the winter, and we have attributed it to costiveness produced by want of water and green food. The name given the disease is exactly indicative of its effect on the animal; producing dislike to food, uneasiness, and a continual inclination to extend the fore and hind feet as far as possible, in the same manner the operation of stretching is performed by a horse or dog. The true remedy or rather preventive, would undoubtedly be a supply of green food; but we have never found anything more necessary than a plentiful supply of salt, to remove the disease at once. The writer in the Cultivator recommends a spoonful of castor oil to be given the sheep, repeating, we presume, the dose, at suitable intervals, till the disease is removed.

TAR FOR SHEEP.

A gentleman who has a large flock of sheep says,

that during the season of grazing he gives his sheep tar, at the rate of a gill a day to every twenty sheep. He puts the tar in troughs, sprinkles a little fine salt over it, and the sheep consume it with eagerness. This preserves them from worms in the head, promotes their health in general, and is thought to be a good specific against the rot.

DISEASE OF HOGS.

Hogs are subject to various diseases; but, according to Laurence, they are not easily doctored. They are subject, he says, to pox or measles, blood-striking, staggers, quincy, indigestion, catarrh, peripneumonia, and inflammation of the lungs, called heavings. When not very sick, pigs will eat, and they will take medicine in their wash. When they will not, there is no help for them. As aperients, cleansers, and alteratives, sulphur, antimony, and madder are our grand specifics, and are truly useful; as cordials and tonics, treacle and strong beer, in warm wash, and good peas and pollard; in the measles, sulphur, &c.; and if the patient require it, give cordials now and then in staggers, bleeding, fresh air, and perhaps nitre; in catarrh a warm bed and warm cordial wash, and the same in quinsy or inflammation of the glands of the throat. If external suppuration appear likely, discharge the matter when ripe, and dress with tar and brandy, or balsam. The heavings, or unsoundness of the lungs in pigs, like the unsoundness of the liver in lambs, is sometimes found to be hereditary. There is no remedy. The disease in pigs is often in consequence of colds from wet lodgings, or hasty feeding in a poor state. In a certain stage it is highly inflammatory, and without remedy. Unction with train oil, and the internal use of it, have been sometimes thought beneficial.

TO PREVENT SICKNESS IN HOGS.

I will give you my experience and opinion on the manner of keeping hogs in health while they are fattening. I have lost in years back a great many hogs, had others sick and languishing, so that they would not fatten, and been obliged to turn them out of the pen. I always observed that my hogs in the pen would eat and chew with eagerness all hard substances, such as peach stones, bones, and every small stone, and that they were particularly fond of coals, such as had by accident got from the fire into their food. I had also observed that when I let a sick hog out of the pen, he would go to eating such things, and even the ground itself. I then thought of trying the experiment, and collected a peck of coals from my casks, and put them into the pen. They were immediately devoured. I gave them more, until my hogs had eaten at least two quarts each. I thought them good, and continued to supply them daily with them. I have since that time (two years ago) fattened more than fifty hogs, and never had a sick one, nor one whose pork was measly or affected with any disease. I believe it to be an effectual remedy for a very serious difficulty with farmers. My neighbours, to whom I have communicated my plan, tried it with the same success, and you may, if you please, give it publicity in your paper.—*Penn. Farmer.*

TO CURE THE SWELLING OF THE THROAT IN HOGS.

In order to contribute to the usefulness of your valuable periodical, and to inform the public what I find from experience to be an infallible cure for a certain disease in hogs, viz. the swelling of the throat, I herewith send you a receipt for the disease, with a desire that you will publish the same in your work, if you deem it of any import, and the same meet your approbation.

Take of molasses one half pint, and a tablespoonful of hog's lard melted; to this add one tablespoonful flour of sulphur; mix well, and drench the hog with it, and nine times out of ten it will be found to have the desired effect. My hogs were affected with this disease during the past year, and I found the above to be effective, when all things else failed.

Farmer's Register.

TO DESTROY VERMIN IN HOGS.

Mix a little tar with grease of any kind sufficient to make the tar thin, then pour it over the hogs when fed sufficiently so as to have them well smeared with the tar. This may be repeated often in the summer and fall, or in good weather. You may give each hog a small tablespoonful of sulphur in their food, or in damp weather have them well sprinkled with strong wood ashes: either of these remedies will prevent or destroy the vermin.

ANOTHER.—Cut a few pods of red pepper in small pieces, and fry them in lard until they change their colour; then mix it with tar and a small quantity of spirits of turpentine, and rub or smear it on the affected parts, and along the back and sides. It will effectually drive away the lice.

TO DESTROY WORMS IN THE KIDNEY OF HOGS.
From the Democrat. (Maine).

MR. EDITOR:—I am induced to send you the following statement, not so much from the importance of this particular case, as from its being a link in the great chain of testimony in favour of a more humane improved treatment of diseased hogs.

In October last, I observed that a thrifty young shoat of mine was weak in the back: he grew worse for several days, until he could scarcely move about, or even get up. At this stage of disease, I commenced feeding him with corn, boiled soft in strong ley, with the addition of a handful of charcoal. This feed was continued four or five days, at which time the hog had to all appearance become as well as ever, and so continues to this time. J. D. HILL.

CURE FOR THE MANGE IN HOGS.

Give them sulphur in their food, and wash them in soap-suds. B. C. LEAVELL.

CURE FOR THE MANGE AND QUINSY IN HOGS.

MESSRS. EDITORS:—During my peregrinations through old "Robertson," a few days since, in conversation with one of its most intelligent citizens (and one of your subscribers too), I was informed of two sovereign remedies for two common diseases to which hogs are liable, to wit: "Mange" and "Quinsy." If you have not already given to your many readers the same or other better remedies for the same diseases, you might do well to give them this, which I am assured has never failed, in many trials, to produce a perfect cure in a short time. The remedy for that most loathsome disease, mange, is simply this:—take the common poke-root, stalks and leaves, and boil a quantity of it until the liquid becomes quite strong, then season with salt, meal, pot-liquor, &c., until it is made palatable to the hog, and he will partake of it and the salad most bountifully. It has been observed, too, that if the hog has ticks on him, they all drop off after the first or second feed; but whether from the liquor getting on him, whilst feeding, or taking it inwardly, is not known. For the quinsy, give the hog tea, made strong of pennyroyal, and seasoned as the poke-juice, with salt, meal, and pot-liquor. It may be repeated for two or three days till relief is given. We have long known that poke-root was a valuable medicine for many diseases incident to domestic animals. We believe a strong tea of poke-root, given frequently, will cure the malignant disease denominated Farcy. It acts upon the skin and the absorbents, and " cleanses the blood."

AGRICULTURIST.

CURE OF MANGE IN DOGS.

To the Editor of the Farmer's Register.—Some years ago, when residing in the upper country, I had a very beautiful and favourite pointer. He became mangy over his whole body, and very much reduced, so that I expected to lose him. I had a friend residing in the neighbourhood who owned a tan-yard. He was kind enough to take my dog for a week or ten days, and dip him in the tan-vat several times each day. He was then rubbed well with a mixture of tanner's oil and tar, and sent home. In the course of a short time the scales began to peel off, and new hair to grow out. He soon became the sleekest and prettiest animal I ever saw, and was never again affected with the disease, or even visited by vermin for a year or two. I often thought, by his playful antics, that he was conscious of his obligations, and wished to express with kindness a gratitude which he felt;

but the obligations were transferred to me, for he lived to afford me many an hour of sport, and many a nice dish of game. The disease is evidently infectious, and those that are subjects of it should not be permitted to consort with those that are not.

I hope the few brief remarks above, may lead to the relief of many a valuable animal for the mutual protection and enjoyment of himself and owner.

W. J. DUPUY.

ANOTHER.—Mix pounded sulphur with common lard, and let the dog eat as much as he pleases; then anoint him well down the middle of his back, and behind his ears, with the balance. Persisted in two or three times, this will certainly effect a cure.

BRIEF HINTS FOR WINTER.
From the Genesee Farmer.

Cattle, and all domestic animals, should commence the winter in good condition. Do not undertake to winter more cattle than you have means of providing for. Let every farmer aim to have next spring, instead of thin, bony, slab-sided, shaggy cattle, fine smooth, round, and healthy ones; and to this end let him spare no pains; and 1st. Let the cattle be well fed. 2d. Let them be fed regularly. 3d. Let them be properly sheltered from the pelting storm. Proper food, and regularity in feeding, will save flesh on the animal's back, and shelter will save the fodder. All domestic animals, in considerable numbers, should be divided into parcels and separated from each other, in order that the weaker may not suffer from the domination of the stronger, nor the diseased from the vigorous.

Farmers who have raised root crops (and all good

farmers have doubtless done so), should cut them up, and mix them with drier food, as meal, chopped hay, straw, or cornstalks, and feed them to cattle or sheep.

Cow-houses and cattle-stables should be kept very clean, and well littered. To allow animals to lie down in the filth, which is sometimes suffered to collect in the stables, is perfectly insufferable.

By using plants of straw, or litter, the consequent quantity of manure will much more than repay the supposed waste of straw, or time to gather trash from the woods to litter stables or cow-pens with.

All stables should be properly ventilated.

Mixing food is generally better than feeding cattle on one substance alone. Cattle will generally eat straw with as much readiness as hay, if it is salted copiously, which may be done by sprinkling brine over it. A great saving is made by cutting not only straw and cornstalks, but hay also.

Sheep, as well as all other domestic animals, should have a constant supply of good water during the winter. They should also be properly sheltered from the storm; for the great point in the secret of keeping them in good condition is to keep them comfortable.

INDEX.

GARDENING.

	Page.		Page.
Apples	89	Orchards, apple	81
Asparagus	13	Okra	31
Artichoke	15	Onions	31
Beans	18	Onions, mode of raising in the town of Wethersfield, Ct.	32
Beets	17	Parsley	36
Borecole	20	Parsnips	35
Brocoli	21	Peach Tree, culture of	78
Cabbage, early	23	Peas, English	37
Cabbage, raising from cuttings	23	Peppers	36
Cabbage, to kill lice on	24	Perry	93
Cabbage, to destroy worms on	24	Plants, soapsuds for watering	89
Carrots	22	Potatoes	38
Cauliflowers	22	Potatoes, another method of raising	38
Celery, solid	24	Potatoes, Irish, mode of preserving	63
Cider, directions for making	90	Potatoes, to improve the quality of	65
Cider, Kerrison's recipe for	92	Potatoes, another	65
Cowkeeping, profits of	95	Potatoes, sweet, successful mode of keeping	61
Cucumbers	26	Potatoes, sweet, another	62
Cucumbers, novel mode of raising	27	Radishes	39
Curled Cress	25	Rhubard, or Pie Plant, to improve the quality of	39
Egg Plant	28	Ruta Baga	44
Fruit Trees	86	Salsify, or Vegetable Oyster	40
Fruit Trees, management of	72	Savory, summer	42
Geological Definitions	94	Seed Corn, on preparing	104
Gherkins	28	Shallots	40
Gourds	29	Spinach	41
Grafting, cement for	89	Spinach, New Zealand	40
Grapes, remedy against mildew	78	Squashes, winter or late running	57
Grain, to correct damaged	60	Steam boiler worth having	98
Hint to Farmers	60	Strawberries	48
Kail	29	Strawberries, observations on the culture of	50
Land, manner of sowing, cultivation, &c.	44	Sugar, corn stalk	99
Lavender, sage, balm, tansey, thyme, rue, rosemary, &c.	30	Tomatoes	55
Leeks	34	Trees, on plugging	87
Lettuce	29		
Manure, Jauffret's mode of manufacturing	102		
Mustard	30		
Nasturtiums	30		

	Page.
Trees, worms in	89
Trees, composition for healing wounds in	89
Turnips, spring	42
Turnips, remedy for destroying the fly	43
Vines	55
Vines, to remove bugs from	60
Vine, the grape, culture of	66
Vine, the grape, another mode	69
Vine, the grape, another	70
Vine, the grape, to prune to advantage	77
Water Melons, directions for the cultivation of	58
Worm, the canker	88
Worm, another	88

COOKERY.

	Page.
Apples, preservation of	156
Apples and pears, dried	160
Attar of roses	177
Beer, to make hop	175
Beer, to make spruce	176
Beer, good, another method	176
Beer tar, for consumption	176
Beer persimmon, to make	177
Beets, to pickle	170
Biscuit, Naples, to make	114
Biscuit, sugar	114
Biscuit, milk	183
Biscuit, butter	184
Blackberry cordial	154
Bread, to make good	107
Bread, excellent without yeast	108
Bread, short way to make old new	108
Bread, soda	109
Bread, dyspepsia	110
Bread, potatoe	111
Bread, rice family	111
Bread, turnip	112
Bread, pumpkin	112
Bread, corn	112
Bread, corn light	113
Bread, another	113
Bunns, Mrs. G.'s famous	122
Butter, apple	152
Cabbage, preservation of	158
Cabbage, to pickle	169
Cake, cider	118
Cake, sponge	119
Cake, another called in France biscuit	184
Cake, pound	120
Cake, Indian pound	183
Cake, cup	183
Cake, potatoe	186
Cake, gingerbread	120
Cake rice, to make	115
Cakes, rice	185
Cakes, rice griddle	116
Cakes, rice Johnny	116
Cakes, another	116
Cakes, Indian meal	116
Cakes, buckwheat	117
Cakes, another	117
Cakes, oyster, corn	117
Cakes, pan	118
Cakes, Washington	118
Cakes, flannel	118
Catsup, tomato	155
Celery sauce for roasted or boiled fowls	149
Cheese, omelet	189
Cherries, to dry	159
Chowder, to make	138
Citron watermelon, to preserve	163
Codfish, how to cook	149
Coffee, improved method of making	151
Coffee, to make good out of rye	151
Corn, to preserve green for boiling	158
Crab-apples, to preserve	165
Crackers, sweet	115
Crackers, dyspepsia	115
Crackers, rice	115
Cranberries, to preserve	165
Cream, substitute for	180

INDEX.

	Page.		Page.
Croquettes	187	Peaches, to brandy	161
Crullers	124	Peaches, to pickle	172
Cucumbers, to pickle	167	Pearl barley, substitute for rice	139
Cucumbers, another	168	Pearl barley, another	140
Cucumbers, another with whiskey and vinegar	168	Peas, green, how to cook	143
		Peas, green, to preserve	158
Cucumbers, stewed	189	Pie, chicken	137
Custard, apple	126	Pie, lobster	190
Custard, plain	126	Pie, oyster	137
Custard, tea	188	Pie, to make a pigeon	137
Doughnuts	124	Pie, to make a mutton	138
Dumpling, apple	127	Pie, to make a pork	138
Dumpling, Norfolk	127	Pie, to make mince	134
Egg-Plant, the purple, or Guinea squash	141	Pie, to make pumpkin	135
		Pie, another	135
Eggs, preservation of	180	Pie, another	135
Eggs, another	181	Pie, to make apple	135
Eggs, another	181	Pie, cranberry	136
Figs, green, to preserve	162	Pie, rhubarb	136
Figs, tomato	163	Pie, sweet potatoe	136
Floating Island	124	Pie, tomato	136
Force-meat balls	146	Pineapple, to preserve	166
Fricassee of fowls	190	Pippins, golden, to preserve	164
Fritters, apple	127	Plumbs and peaches, to keep fresh through the year	158
Fritters, bread	187		
Gherkins, to pickle	171	Pork, frying	148
Gingerbread, soft, very nice	120	Potatoes, directions for boiling	150
Gingerbread, common	121	Potatoes, another	150
Grapes, to pickle	171	Potatoes, frozen	159
Grapes, to preserve	165	Potatoe flour	189
Grapes, to preserve plums and, in a fresh state	157	Pudding, apple	128
		Pudding, Indian	128
Hash, a fine	191	Pudding, plain Indian baked	128
Jam, raspberry	155	Pudding, rich Indian baked	129
Jelly, apple	153	Pudding, Indian boiled	129
Jelly, calf's feet	144	Pudding, green corn	129
Jelly, peach	153	Pudding, potatoe	130
Jelly, red or black currant	154	Pudding, sweet potatoe	130
Jelly, rice	154	Pudding, pumpkin	130
Jumbles	121	Pudding, carrot	130
Kisses	125	Pudding, to make pap	131
Marguerites	187	Pudding, transparent	131
Meat, cooking	146	Pudding, to make a bath	131
Mead, to make	175	Pudding, quaking	131
Melon-Mangoes, to pickle	170	Pudding, bread	132
Metheglin, to make	175	Pudding, rich bread and butter	132
Milk, to preserve	179	Pudding, plum	132
Molasses, apple	151	Pudding, a Carolina rice	133
Muffins, soft	124	Pudding, another	133
Mutton, with oysters	191	Pudding, rules to be observed in making a	133
Onions, to pickle	169		
Oysters, to pickle	166	Pudding, turkey	190
Peaches, dried	160	Puffs, rice	116

400 INDEX.

	Page.		Page.
Purlow	139	Sour krout, to pickle	172
Pumpkins, to preserve in a fresh state	158	Starch, to make	178
		Strawberries, to preserve in wine	162
Quinces, to preserve whole	161		
Raspberries, to preserve	162	Strawberries, to preserve whole	162
Rice milk for dessert	126	Sugar, to clarify	166
Rice, how to boil	140	Sweetmeats, to make peach	161
Rissoles	188	Syrup, orange	155
Rolls	123	Tomato, spiced	156
Rusk	122	Tomato, to preserve in a fresh state	156
Rusk, corn meal	123		
Receipts for housekeeper's	181	Tomato, to pickle	169
Salad, washing of	151	Vinegar, to make	178
Salsify, or vegetable oyster	140	Wafers	186
Salsify, another	140	Wafers, Graham	115
Sauce, bread	192	Wafers, rice	115
Sauce, melted butter	194	Walnuts, to pickle	167
Sausage, to make	145	Wine, to make currant	173
Sausage, another	145	Wine, parsnip	173
Sausage, Oxford	145	Wine, ginger	174
Soda for washing	178	Wine, orange	174
Soup, okra	141	Wine and cider, mode of refining	178
Soup, beef	193		
Soup, to make calf's head	143	Yeast, milk	114
Soup, oyster	193	Yeast for bread	113
Soup, pea	192	Yeast, another	113
Soup, green pea	192		

DOMESTIC DEPARTMENT.

	Page.		Page.
Ants, red, to destroy	242	Calicos, to wash well	238
Bacon, to cure	222	Candles, to make dip	229
Bed-bugs	242	Candles, a new way to make	231
Beef, to preserve tender	225	Capons, to make	204
Bees, hunting	213	Cask, to stop leak in	261
Bees, taking hives without destroying the	213	Cattle, estimating weight of	271
		Cement for mending crockery	245
Bee-house, plan of	210	Cement, japan or rice glue	256
Beeswax, to bleach	239	Chickens, to fatten fowls and	202
Blacking	253	Chickens, to cure gaps in	203
Block-tin and pewter, method of cleaning	244	China, Chinese method of mending	245
Bottles, decanters, &c. to clean	244	Cockroaches, to destroy	243
Browning steel or iron	263	Composition to make common wood resemble mahogany	249
Butter, making	215		
Butter, patent	217	Composition, useful	250
Butter, strong	217	Composition to defend the roof of a house from the weather and fire	251
Butter, salting	218		
Butter, packing	220		

INDEX. 401

	Page.
Composition for preserving farmer's utensils	251
Composition to preserve boots and shoes	253
Corn, measuring	266
Crows, how to kill	268
Crows, to prevent pulling up corn	269
Eggs and poultry	199
Eggs, hen's	202
Eggs, to prevent dogs from sucking	204
Fence posts	264
Fish ponds	215
Fleas, to prevent	242
Flies, to destroy	243
Flies, to prevent sitting on pictures	243
Glass, to remove panes of	246
Grease for wheel axles	262
Hams, to cure	224
Hamborough pickle	225
Harness, preservation of	252
How to get a tight ring of a finger	245
Ice-house and dairy, plan of	205
Ice-house, a portable	209
Ink-spots, to remove	238
Ink spots, to remove from linen	238
Ink or wine, to take out	238
Ink, permanent, for marking	259
Ink, marking or durable	259
Ink, to make black	260
Ink, black, improved composition of	260
Ink, red	261
Ink, printer's, how to prepare	261
Interest, to calculate	267
Iron-mould, to remove	238
Knives and forks, to clean	247
Lamps, to prevent smoking	250
Linen, to take mildew out of	250
Mattrass, how to make a	210
Meat, to preserve fresh	225
Meat, to restore tainted	226
Meat, fish, &c., to sweeten	226
Mortar, a valuable, to prevent soot from accumulating in chimneys	250
Moths, to prevent	239
Moulding, to prevent	247
Nails, to preserve from rust	262
Paste	246
Paint, a cheap white	258

	Page.
Paint, to clean	246
Paint, a cheap green	259
Pictures, to clean	247
Pig-troughs	264
Poke-berry dye	234
Polish for dining tables	249
Pork, curing	221
Rats, to destroy	241
Rats and mice, to expel	241
Razors, composition for	248
Scarecrows	269
Sheepskins, to cure with the wool on	273
Shoes, to prevent taking in water	254
Silk, to take stains out of	236
Silk, woollen, &c., to cleanse	235
Silk, to take grease out of	237
Silk, to wash	237
Silk, to take spots out of, &c.	236
Soap, to make soft	227
Soap, to make hard	228
Soap, to make cold	228
Soap, a simple method	229
Smoky chimneys	250
Stains by fruit, to remove	238
To dye cotton yarn	231
To color green	232
To color red	232
To dye red	233
To dye crimson	233
To dye pink	234
To color yellow	234
To color flannel	234
To color nankeen	234
To clean silk stockings	236
To take mildew out of linen	236
To take stains out of silk	236
To take spots out of silk, linen, &c.	236
To extract a glass stopper	246
Turkeys, method of rearing	197
Varnish, japan, copal	255
Water, to purify	240
Wasps, effective method to kill	267
Window sashes, to keep up	248
White-wash, to make	257
White-wash, to make a brilliant stucco	257
White-wash, to make a cheap paint or	257
Wolves and crows, to destroy	270
Wood, to polish	248
Writings, old, to revive	247

DISEASES OF MAN.

	Page.		Page.
Arsenic, remedy for	299	Jaundice, cure for	310
Asthma, cure for	308	Life, restoring, to the apparently drowned	281
Bathing	277		
Bleeding at the nose	283	Life, animal	281
Blood to stop	282	Measles, cure for	310
Burns, remedy for	303	Ointment, Burdon's excellent	283
Cancer, cure for	291	Opodeldoc, to make	283
Cancer, another	311	Palsy, cure for	310
Cholera morbus, cure for	288	Piles, cure for	296
Cough, cure for	308	Poison, onions an antidote for	287
Cough, cold or, cure for	318	Poison by arsenic, antidote for	288
Colic, cure for	309	Poison, cure for	313
Colds, remedy for	307	Polypus in the nose, cure for	293
Consumption, cure for	316	Remedy in case of swallowing pins, fish bones, &c.	282
Corns, cure for	299		
Costiveness, cure for	280	Rhumatism, cure for	301
Cramp in the stomach	300	Ringworm	305
Croup, cure for	297	Salt rheum, cure for	290
Deafness, cure for	300	Slippery-elm, powder of	284
Dropsy, cure for	294	Spasms, cure for	289
Dysentery, cure for	297	Strengthening plaster	303
Earache, cure for	305	Summer complaint, cure for	299
Eye, films on, remedy for	306	Teeth, to cleanse	282
Eye-water, cure for sore eyes	306	Tetter, cure for	292
Eye-water, another, for chronic sore eyes	306	Thrush, cure for	299
		Throat, sore, cure for	309
Felon, cure for	292	Throat, putrid sore, cure for	309
Fever and ague, cure for	312	Toothache, Dr. Blake's remedy for	305
Fever, scarlet, cure for	315		
Fever, scarlet, prevention of	316	Urine, suppression of	280
Food, time required to digest	279	Urine, to promote	280
Frost-bitten	283	Vomiting, to stop	283
Gangrene	289	Viper, cure for the bite of	284
Gestation	282	Wart, cancer, cure for	291
Gout, cure for	301	Warts, cure for	300
Gravel, cure for	295	Wasp or bee, cure for sting of	291
Heart-burn, cure for	310	Wen, cure for	291
Hydrophobia, cure for	287	White swelling, cure for	310
Indigestion remedy for	280	Whooping cough, cure for	308
Influenza, cure for	309	Women's breasts	303
Itch, cure for	293	Worms, cure for	298

DISEASES OF BEASTS.

	Page.		Page.
Blisters	326	Calves, diseases of	376
Botts, remedy for	361	Cattle, to kill lice on	365
Brief Hints for Winter	394	Cattle, to destroy vermin on,	365

INDEX. 403

Cattle, to cure the mange in,	366	Horses, &c., swellings on	324
Cattle, how to relieve choked	370	Horses, &c., King's oil for curing wounds on	324
Cattle, hoven	371	Horses, cracks in the heels, or wounds in	325
Clyster, or Glyster	327		
Cows, remedy for swelled or snarled bags in	373	Horses, lost appetite in	325
Colic, or Gripes	329	Horses, mash for	325
Diseases and treatment of Cattle	364	Horses, cure for scours in	328
		Horses, malander in	335
Disease commonly called the hollow horn	364	Horses, remedy for heaves in	335
		Horses, cure for cough in	335
Distemper in Cattle	364	Horses, thumps in	337
Dogs, cure for mange in	393	Horses, wind-galls in	337
Farcy	346	Horses, sitfast on	338
Farrier, curious case of a	326	Horses, poll evil, or fistula in	341
Fistula	345	Horses, big head in	354
Glanders	353	Horses, gravel in the hoofs of	357
Gravel, stone or, in the bladder	358	Horses, hide-bound	259
		Lampass	355
Hogs, diseases of	389	Lice, to kill, on horses, cows and hogs	364
Hogs, to prevent sickness in	390		
Hogs, to cure swelling of the throat in	390	Lockjaw	356
		Murrain	374
Hogs, to destroy vermin on	391	Murrain, bloody, cure for	374
Hogs, to destroy worms in the kidneys of	391	Murrain and yellow water, cure for	375
Hogs, cure for the mange and quinsy in	392	Ringbone	349
		Salt for cattle	376
Hogs, cure for the mange in	391	Scours in calves, cure for	376
Hoof Ail	366	Scratches	339
Hooks or Haws	355	Sheep, age of	322
Horn distemper, or horn-ail	366	Sheep, poisoned, cure for	376
Horse, a broken-winded	336	Sheep, diseases of	377
Horses, how to form a judgment of the age of	321	Sheep, tar for	388
		Spavin	351
Horses, to prevent being teased by flies	322	Splint	350
		Staggers	343
Horses, sore tongue in	322	Staggers, blind	344
Horses, colic in	329	Strains	348
Horses, liniment for the galled backs of	323	String halt	350
		Swiney	353
Horses, saddle-galls on	323	Yellow water	360
Horses, founder in	332		

CPSIA information can be obtained
at www.ICGtesting.com
Printed in the USA
JSHW050749230921
18866JS00008B/1